For Reference

Not to be taken from this room

D1573104

ATLAS OF FORENSIC
HISTOPATHOLOGY

GRACE LIBRARY CARLOW UNIVERSITY
PITTSBURGH PA 15213

ATLAS OF FORENSIC HISTOPATHOLOGY

Peter M. Cummings, M.D.

*Medical Examiner and Director of Forensic Neuropathology, Office of the
Chief Medical Examiner Commonwealth of Massachusetts, Boston, MA, USA.*

Darin P. Trelka, M.D., Ph.D.

*Associate Medical Examiner, Broward County Medical
Examiner and Trauma Services, FL, USA.*

Kimberley M. Springer, M.D.

*Medical Examiner, Office of the Chief Medical Examiner Commonwealth of
Massachusetts, Boston, MA, USA.*

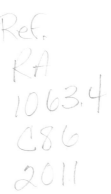

Ref.
RA
1063.4
C86
2011

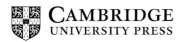

CAMBRIDGE
UNIVERSITY PRESS

CATALOGUED

CAMBRIDGE UNIVERSITY PRESS
Cambridge, New York, Melbourne, Madrid, Cape Town, Singapore,
São Paulo, Delhi, Dubai, Tokyo, Mexico City

Cambridge University Press
The Edinburgh Building, Cambridge CB2 8RU, UK

Published in the the United States of America by Cambridge University Press, New York

www.cambridge.org
Information on this title: www.cambridge.org/9780521110891

© Cambridge University Press 2011

This publication is in copyright. Subject to statutory exception
and to the provisions of relevant collective licensing agreements,
no reproduction of any part may take place without the written
permission of Cambridge University Press.

First published 2011

Printed in the United Kingdom at the University Press, Cambridge

A catalog record for this publication is available from the British Library

Library of Congress Cataloging in Publication data
Cummings, Peter M., 1971–
    Atlas of forensic histopathology / Peter M. Cummings, Darin P. Trelka, Kimberley M. Springer.
        p. ; cm.
    Includes bibliographical references and index.
    ISBN 978-0-521-11089-1 (hardback)
    1. Forensic pathology–Atlases.   2. Histology, Pathological–Atlases.   I. Trelka, Darin P.
    II. Springer, Kimberley M.   III. Title.
    [DNLM: 1. Forensic Pathology–Atlases. W 617]
    RA1063.4.C86 2011
    614´.1–dc22   2010034898

ISBN 978-0-521-11089-1 Hardback

Cambridge University Press has no responsibility for the persistence or
accuracy of URLs for external or third-party internet websites referred to in
this publication, and does not guarantee that any content on such websites is,
or will remain, accurate or appropriate.

All material contained within the CD-ROM is protected by copyright and other
intellectual property laws. The customer acquires only the right to use the CD-ROM
and does not acquire any other rights, express or implied, unless these are stated
explicitly in a separate licence.

To the extent permitted by applicable law, Cambridge University Press is not liable for
direct damages or loss of any kind resulting from the use of this product or from errors
or faults contained in it, and in every case Cambridge University Press's liability shall
be limited to the amount actually paid by the customer for the product.

Every effort has been made in preparing this book to provide accurate and up-to-date
information which is in accord with accepted standards and practice at the time of publication.
Although case histories are drawn from actual cases, every effort has been made to disguise the
identities of the individuals involved. Nevertheless, the authors, editors and publishers can
make no warranties that the information contained herein is totally free from error, not least
because clinical standards are constantly changing through research and regulation. The authors,
editors, and publishers therefore disclaim all liability for direct or consequential damages resulting
from the use of material contained in this book. Readers are strongly advised to pay careful attention
to information provided by the manufacturer of any drugs or equipment that they plan to use.

To mom and dad, I miss you both.

To Sarah and Fionn, thank you for all the love and support (and for the occasional brief moments of quiet while I tried to finish this thing).

To my big sis Shawna, for all the years of believing I could, even when I had doubts.

To Dr. John Butt, Former Chief Medical Examiner of Nova Scotia. Without you, none of this would have happened. Thank you for introducing me to the amazing world of forensic pathology!

Peter Cummings

To my parents for providing me everything and asking nothing in return.

To my wife and daughter for loving and supporting me through the journey and for always reminding me what is important.

To Ted, Melissa, Chris, Christian, Ian, Joe, Mark, Kevin and Grant, who have influenced my career more than you know.

To Paul and Pete for introducing me to the wonder of forensics.

To the Office of the Chief Medical Examiner of the Commonwealth of Virginia for showing all of us "the way."

To the Cuyahoga County Coroner's Office for some of the source materials for this book.

To Steve for the great micrographs, and the opportunity.

To all the trainees in forensic pathology, who must remember the oft quoted adage, "The eye can't see what the mind doesn't know."

Finally, to Dr. Marcella Fierro for instilling in me the need to "take *the word* out."

Darin Trelka

To Michele, thanks for being my favorite lady.

To Lisa, thanks for letting me work on this, even when it annoyed you.

To all past, present, and future Forensic Pathology Fellows – enjoy!

Kimberley Springer

CONTENTS

FOREWORD

Histopathology examination is the daily bread and butter of the general or special-expertise pathologist. However, for many years histopathology had been under-evaluated in many Medical Examiners' and Coroners' Offices here in the USA, and had not been treated much better in the remainder of the world. Nevertheless, in recent decades there has been an increased awareness of the central importance of forensic microscopy in many forensic cases, and the number of histopathology books has increased significantly. However, there are still very few atlases of forensic pathology and by publishing their *Atlas of Forensic Histopathology*, Drs. Cummings, Trelka and Springer have made a highly valuable contribution to forensic medicine. All three authors are experienced and highly regarded Medical Examiners, with an aggregate experience of decades in forensic histopathology. While textbooks of forensic histopathology are valuable, the number of illustrative photos included is always much less than that presented in a microscopy atlas. In the forensic pathology world, as much as in the world at large, a picture is better evidence than a thousand words. Besides presenting a wealth of forensic microscopic illustrations, the authors of this atlas have eminently succeeded in selecting a wide spectrum of color illustrations from both common and difficult type of cases, including the challenging issues of aging of natural, chemical, and traumatic injuries. The legends to the illustrations are very clear and are accompanied by guiding tables of differential diagnoses and time-related pathogenetic changes. The atlas is valuable both to the novice forensic pathologist and to the experienced one, facing a difficult case or in need of supportive or documentary evidence.

The Atlas of Forensic Histopathology by Cummings, Trelka and Springer is an effective and easy-to-use professional tool which should be available in every forensic library.

Joshua A. Perper M.D., L.L.B., M.Sc
Director and Chief Medical Examiner
Broward County Office of Medical Examiner and Trauma Services
Fort Lauderdale, Florida, USA

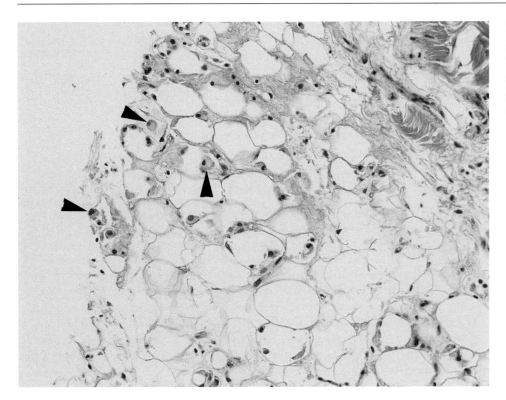

Figure 1.2B. Section of subdermal adipose tissue with numerous foamy macrophages (arrow heads), many of which are visible with stainable iron.

Table 1.1 Contusion ageing.

Time interval	Histologic appearance
< 4 hours	- No distinct signs of inflammation - Histological distinction between antemortem and postmortem skin wounds not possible. (Caveat: neutrophilic infiltrates have been reported to appear within 20–30 minutes [1])
4–12 hours	**4 hours**: Some perivascular neutrophils **8–12 hours**: Neutrophils, macrophages, and fibroblasts form a distinct peripheral wound zone. (neutrophils >> macrophages)
12–48 hours	**16–24 hours**: Macrophage infiltrate increases. (macrophages >> neutrophils) **24 hours**: Neutrophils and fibrin deposition at maximum and remain for 2–3 days Cut edge of epidermis shows cytoplasmic processes **24–48 hours**: Epidermis migrates from the edge toward the center of the wound **32 hours**: Necrosis is apparent in central wound zone **48 hours**: Macrophages reach maximum in peripheral wound zone
2–4 days	**2–4 days**: Fibroblasts migrate into wound periphery. Stainable hemosiderin apparent [1][3] **3 days**: Epithelialization of small wounds becomes complete and its stratification is thicker than surrounding epithelium **3–4 days**: Angiogenesis occurs

continued on next page

Table 1.1 *continued*

Time interval	Histologic appearance
4–8 days	**4 days**: New collagen laid down **4–5 days**: Ingrowth of new capillaries, which continues until day 8 **6 days**: Lymphocytes at maximum in peripheral zone **4–8 days**: Copious stainable hemosiderin
8–12 days	- Decrease in number of inflammatory cells, fibroblasts, and capillaries - Increase in the number and size of collagen fibers - Hematoidin becomes apparent
>12 days	- Definite regression of cellular activity in both epidermis and dermis. Vascularity of dermis decreases. Collagen fibers restored and begin to mature and shrink. Epithelium shows definite basement membrane

Table adapted from [2]. Speed of changes are different in different tissues, even in contralateral sites of the same person [3]. Gross and histologic "contusions", or pseudo-contusions, *can* appear after death [1], especially when there is increasing pressure in local vasculature with subsequent rupture and passive extravasation into the surrounding tissues. In these post-mortem pseudo-contusions, there is no inflammatory "vital reaction" seen histologically; however, "the lack of a vital reaction does not imply that the injury occurred postmortem" [1]. Like all things in forensics, these injuries must be correlated with investigatory and gross anatomic findings.

Source:

[1] Langlois, N.E.I., The science behind the quest to determine the age of bruises – a review of the English language literature. *Forensic Sci Med Pathol*, **3** (2007), 241–251.

[2] Raekallio, J., Histologic estimation of the age of injuries. In Perper, J.A., and Wecht, C.H., eds., *Microscopic Diagnosis in Forensic Pathology*. Springfield, IL: Charles C. Thomas, (1980), pp. 3–16.

[3] Vanezis, P.,Interpreting bruises at necropsy. *J Clin Pathol*, **54** (2001), 348–355.

Brain

Subarachnoid hemorrhage dating

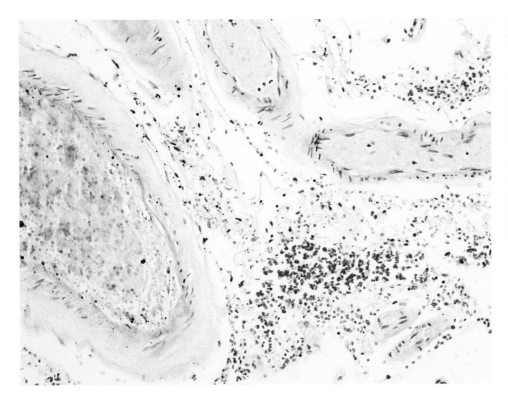

Figure 1.3. Subarachnoid hemorrhage. There is acute hemorrhage in the subarachnoid space. Notice there is no acute inflammatory response and the red blood cell cytoplasmic borders are intact. The age of this lesion is best estimated as less than one hour. After one to four hours neutrophils appear. After four hours the red blood cells begin to lyse.

Table 1.2 Microscopic dating of subarachnoid hemorrhages.

<1 hour	-	Fresh blood in subarachnoid space
1 to 4 hours	-	Occasional neutrophils seen
	-	Some red blood cells begin to break down
	-	Red blood cells begin to creep down the Virchow–Robin spaces
4 to 12 hours	-	Increased neutrophils
	-	Perivascular lymphocytes
	-	Rare macrophages
12 to 24 hours	-	Hemosiderin and fibrin
	-	Increased numbers of lymphocytes and macrophages
24 to 48 hours	-	Increased neutrophils and macrophages
	-	Definite hemosiderin deposition
Up to 3 days	-	Peak neutrophilic infiltrate
Up to 5 days	-	Laking of red blood cells
	-	Increased lymphocytes
	-	Intense fibrin deposition separating islands of red blood cells
	-	Early collagen formation

continued on next page

Table 1.2 *continued*

Up to 1 week	-	Hemosiderin-laden macrophages
	-	Neutrophils fade away
	-	Some intact red blood cells remain
Up to 10 days	-	Fibrosis
	-	Breakdown of red blood cells nears completion (this can take up to 20 days)
Up to 2 weeks	-	Continued break down of red blood cells
	-	Macrophages with hematoidin
	-	Increased organization with additional fibrin, collagen and phagocytosis
Up to 4 weeks	-	Rebleeding
	-	Meningeal reactive changes
	-	Variable amounts of mixed inflammatory cells
After 1 month	-	Macrophages and hemosiderin still present sometimes for years

Subdural hematoma dating

Figure 1.4. Normal baby dura. This section of dura was taken at a site distant from the superior sagittal sinus. If the section is taken too close to the sagittal sinus the intradural blood normally found at that site could be confused with a subdural hemorrhage (compare with Figure 1.5).

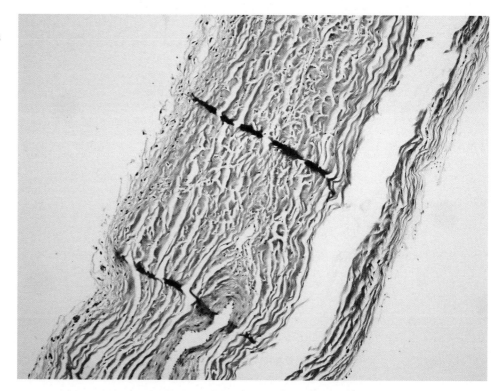

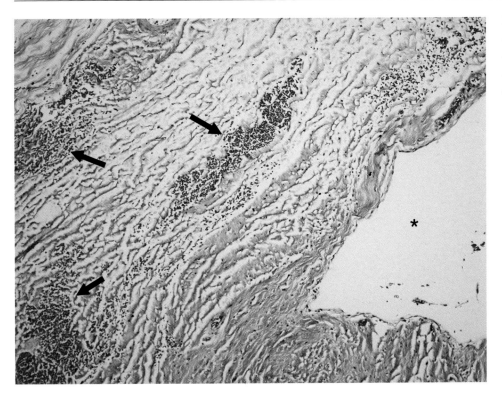

Figure 1.5. Normal baby dura. This section is taken close to the superior sagittal sinus (asterisk). Note the foci of acute hemorrhage (arrows) (compare with Figure 1.4).

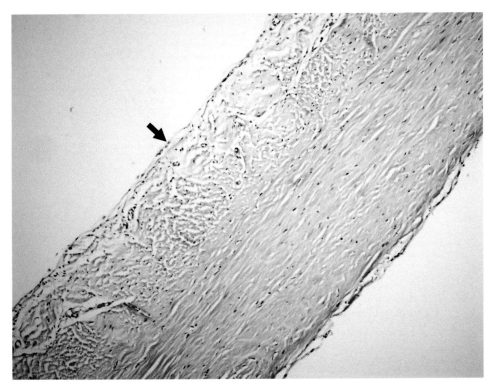

Figure 1.6. Normal adult dura. The meningeal artery designates the periosteal side of the dura (not seen in this section). The dura is comprised of dense fibrotic tissue with sparse spindle-shaped cells. There are small capillaries on the inside of the dura. The thin single-cell layer represents the dura border cells (arrow) that are in contact with the arachnoid barrier cells. This region is the origin of subdural hemorrhages.

Figure 1.7. Acute subdural hemorrhage: 24 to 48 hours. There is acute hemorrhage with fibrin infiltration (arrow). A number of neutrophils are seen and are greater in number close to the dura–hemorrhage interface (arrowheads). Notice the red blood cells are intact.

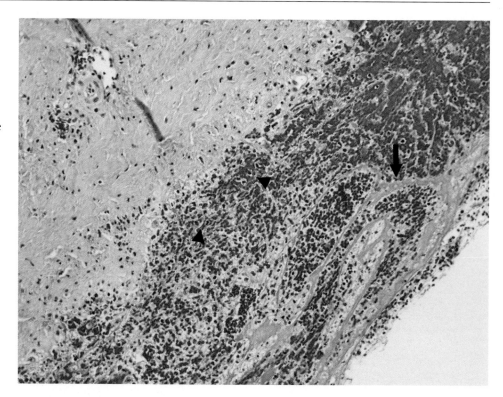

Figure 1.8A. Subdural hematoma: 3 to 4 days. The meningeal artery designates the periosteal side of the dura (arrow head). There is a fibroblast layer forming at the clot–dura interface that is beginning to creep into the hemorrhage (asterisk). Notice the small- caliber blood vessels characteristic of neovascularization (arrow). The red blood cells have begun to lose their distinct cytoplasmic borders as they begin to degenerate. A higher magnification of this same region can be seen in Figure 1.8B.

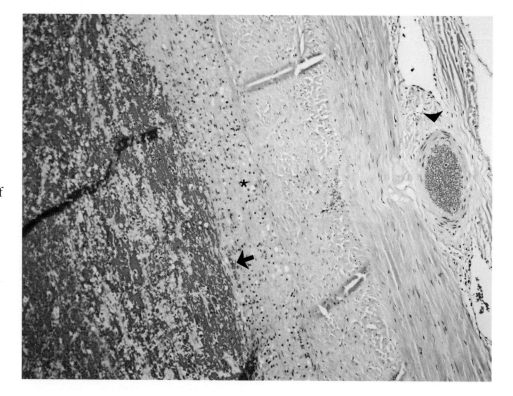

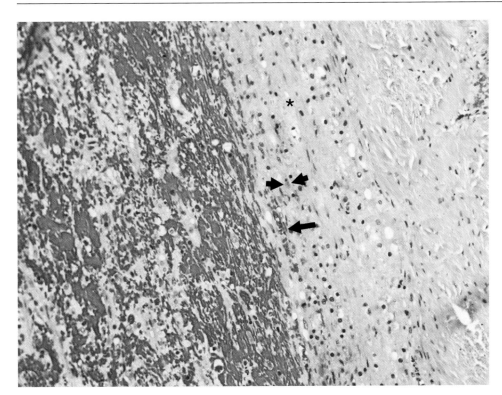

Figure 1.8B. At this level of magnification hemosiderin can be seen (double arrow). There is a fibroblast layer forming at the clot–dural interface that is beginning to creep into the hemorrhage (asterisk). Notice the small-caliber blood vessels characteristic of neovascularization (arrow).

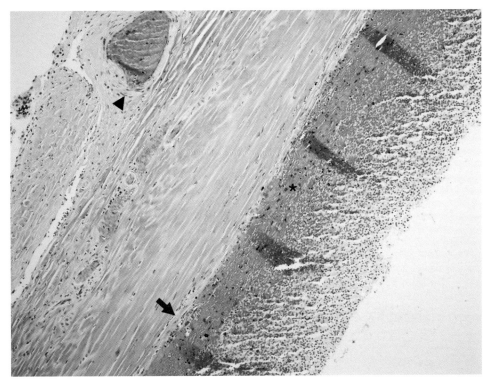

Figure 1.9. Subdural hematoma: 3 to 4 days. The meningeal artery designates the periosteal side (arrow head). There is acute hemorrhage on the subdural side of the dura. There is an early proliferation of fibroblasts, which is forming a layer approximately two cells thick (arrow). Notice the scant fibroblastic infiltrate into the area of hemorrhage (also seen under the arrow). Also, the red blood cells are intact and there is rare hemosiderin deposition (asterisk).

Figure 1.10. Subdural hematoma: 7 days. The fibroblast layer is very thick (between arrows), greater than ten cells in thickness, and there is some migration into the clot (asterisk). Macrophages are present and some contain hemosiderin (arrowhead). The red blood cells have become pale and have lost their distinct cellular borders.

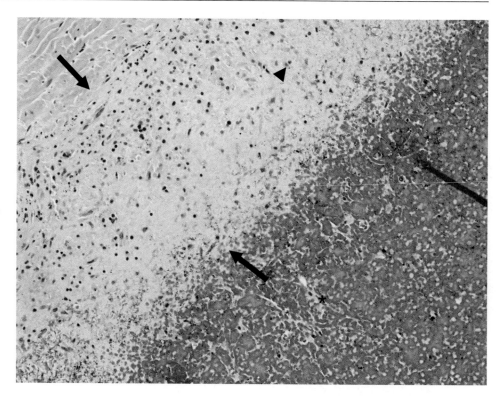

Figure 1.11A. Subdural hematoma: 2 to 3 weeks. The thickness of the neomembrane is close to that of the native dura. Also note the fragment of DuraGel®present at one end of the section (double arrowhead).

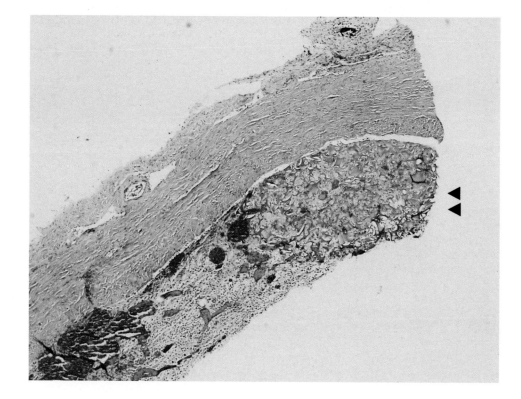

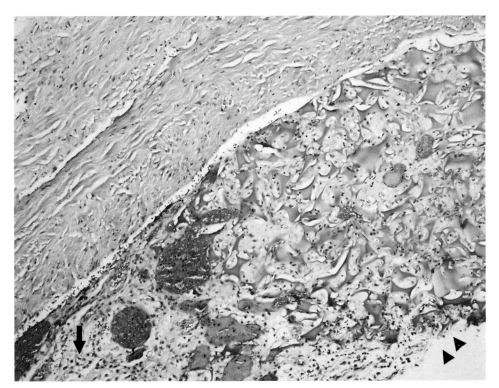

Figure 1.11B. The regions of interest are seen at higher magnification of Figure 1.11A. All of the red blood cells have been absorbed. Giant capillaries are easily seen and there are numerous hemosiderin-laden macrophages present (arrow). Also note the fragment of DuraGel® present at one end of the section (double arrowhead).

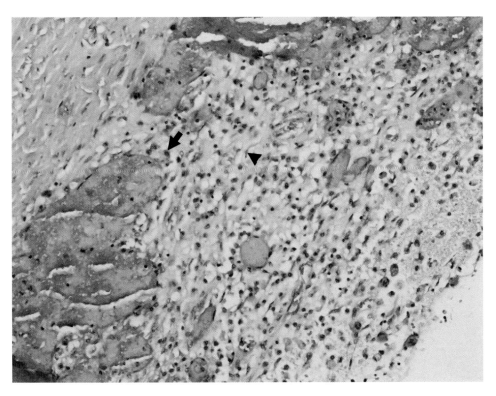

Figure 1.11C. The regions of interest are seen at higher magnification of Figure 1.11A. There are numerous hemosiderin-laden macrophages present (arrow). Fibroblasts, which appear as wavy-looking cells, are beginning to lay down collagen (arrowhead).

Figure 1.12. Subdural hematoma: 3 weeks. There are prominent large capillaries with laking and breakdown of red blood cells. There is a focus of fresh hemorrhage (asterisk). The fibroblastic layer is loosely arranged (between arrowheads) and there is extensive vascular proliferation within the clot that is near the top right-hand side of the photograph. Also present are rare macrophages.

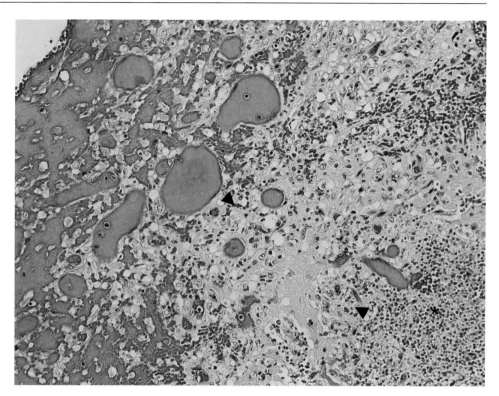

Figure 1.13. Subdural hematoma: various ages. There is a thin collagenized neomembrane (between arrows) representing a remote lesion. There are large-caliber, dilated capillaries (single arrowhead) and some collagen deposits (double arrowheads) also present, suggesting a more recent bleed that is approximately 2 weeks old. Note the acute hemorrhage (double asterisk): this also represents a more recent bleed, probably hours, as there is no inflammatory infiltrate and no fibrin. The neomembrane will thicken to a varying degree, usually to equal the thickness of the dura, over 2 to 3 months.

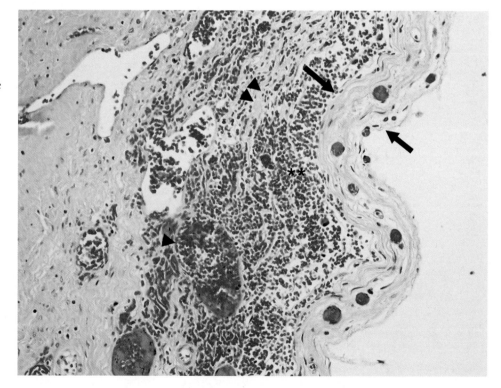

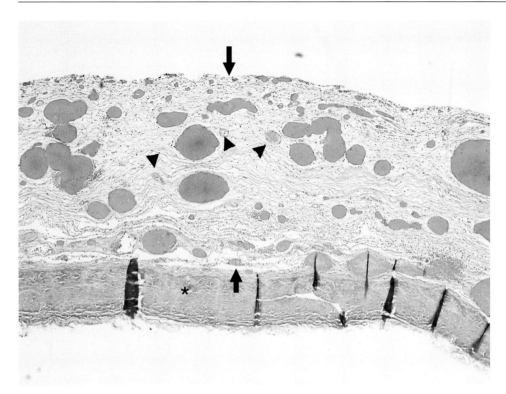

Figure 1.14. Subdural hematoma: 1 to 2 months. The neomembrane (between arrows) is close to twice the thickness of the native dura (asterisk). There are few, if any, red blood cells. Large, dilated capillaries are prominent. Also present are scattered arteries (arrowheads).

Table 1.3 Microscopic dating of subdural hemorrhages.

> 24 hours	-	Intact red blood cells
	-	Some fibrin between the dura and the hemorrhage
24 to 48 hours	-	Increased fibrin deposition
	-	Neutrophils invade hemorrhage
	-	Proliferation of fibroblasts at the interface of the dura and hemorrhage
48 to 72 hours	-	Increased presence of the above
	-	Endothelial proliferation
3 to 5 days	-	Macrophages appear
	-	Early red blood cell breakdown
	-	Neomembrane is 3 to 4 cells thick closer to day 3
	-	Neomembrane will be up to 7 cells thick closer to day 5
5 to 10 days	-	Newly formed capillaries enter the hemorrhage
	-	Laking of red blood cells
	-	Neomembrane is up to 15 cells thick close to day 10
Up to 14 days	-	Hemosiderin-laden macrophages
	-	Neomembrane thickness can be up to twice that of the native dura
	-	Hugely dilated capillaries
Up to 21 days	-	Hemorrhage is absorbed with rare red blood cells remaining
	-	More obvious vascular proliferation
	-	Neomembrane is mostly loosely arranged fibrovascular tissue

continued on next page

Table 1.3 *continued*

Up to 1 month	- Neomembrane is approximately the thickness of the dura
	- Collagen is deposited
	- Formation of arteries
Up to 6 months	- Rare hemosiderin-laden macrophages
	- Fusion of neomembrane and dura
	- Rare blood vessels
Up to 1 year	- Thin neomembrane that is difficult to distinguish from native dura
	- Hemosiderin-laden macrophages still present

Source:

[1] Lindenberg, R.,Trauma of the meninges and brain. In Minckler, J., ed. *Pathology of the Nervous System*. New York: McGraw–Hill, **2** (1971), pp. 1705–1765.

[2] McCormick, W.F., Pathology of closed head injury. In Wilkins, R.H., *et al.*, eds. *Neurosurgery*. New York: McGraw-Hill (1985), pp. 1544–1570.

Cerebral contusion dating

Figure 1.15A. Acute cortical contusion. There is acute hemorrhage at the crest of the gyrus. The red blood cells have intact cytoplasmic borders and there is no inflammatory response. There is edema manifested by the clear spaces around neurons. However, one must be cautious in identifying edema in postmortem specimens, given that there is the potential for autolytic and histologic processing artifact.

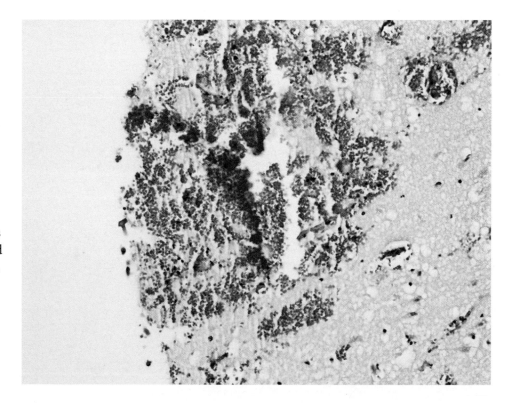

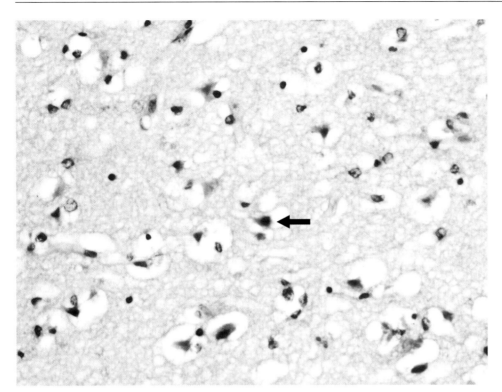

Figure 1.15B. The neurons are demonstrating degenerative changes such as pyknosis and increased eosinophilia, which are most likely the result of trauma and not hypoxia (arrow).

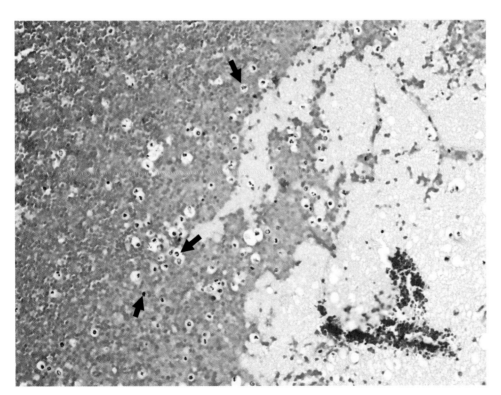

Figure 1.16. Acute cortical contusion: 24 to 72 hours. There is acute hemorrhage accompanied by a mild acute inflammatory infiltrate. Some of the red blood cells are beginning to lose their cytoplasmic borders while others are intact but pale (arrows).

Figure 1.17. Acute cortical contusion: 3 to 5 days. There is acute hemorrhage with some intact red blood cells and some areas of red blood cell pallor with loss of contour. Neutrophils are prominent (arrowheads) with occasional macrophages (arrows). Endothelial proliferation with early neovascularization is also present (asterisk). Notice the enlarged, cleared-out nuclei of the endothelial cells.

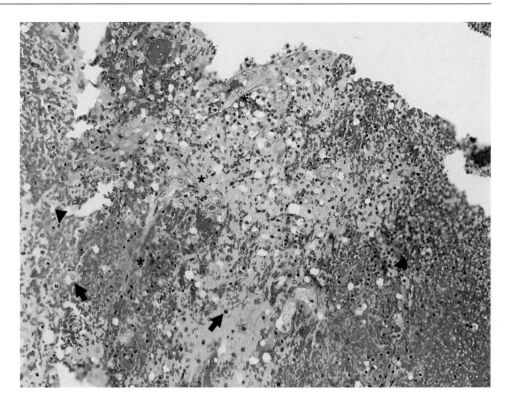

Figure 1.18. Remote cortical contusion. There is a gliotic cyst located at the crest of the gyrus. This is an important feature that distinguishes a contusion from an infarct, where infarcts tend to involve the depth of a sulcus. This contusion is best characterized as months old as there is an intense gliotic reaction and hemosiderin deposition, and well-formed capillaries. Hemosiderin and hemosiderin-laden macrophages can persist for decades (asterisk). Also note the reactive meningeal cells forming whorls (arrows). Arrowheads identify astrocytes and hash marks denote newly forming capillaries.

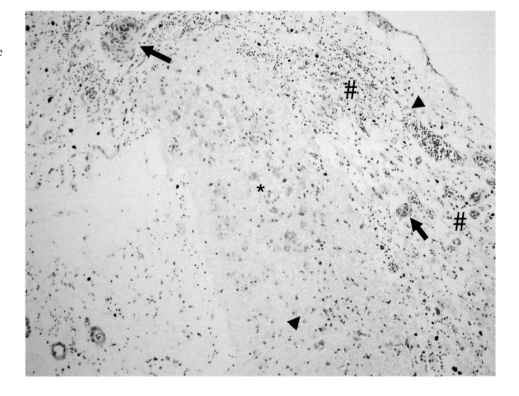

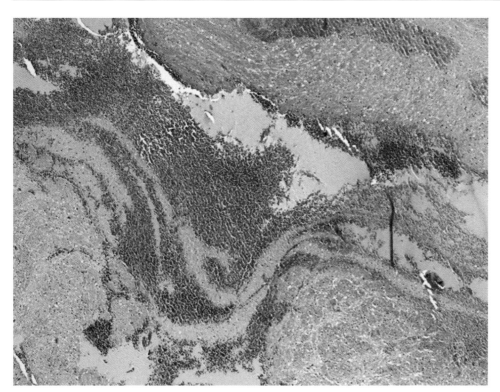

Figure 1.19. Pontine avulsion. There are multiple foci of acute intraparenchymal hemorrhage. This can be differentiated from removal artifact if the pathologist carefully watches the brain removal.

Table 1.4 Microscopic dating of cerebral contusions.

>1 hour	-	Edema
	-	Subarachnoid hemorrhage with hemorrhage into Virchow–Robin space
	-	Hyper-eosinophilic ("red") neurons approximating the lesion
1 to 3 hours	-	Neutrophils begin to enter the parenchyma
	-	Increased acute hemorrhage
3 to 6 hours	-	Increased neutrophilic infiltration
	-	Neuronal encrustation
6 to 12 hours	-	Increased intensity of above
	-	Intense edema with vascular congestion
12 to 24 hours	-	Endothelial cell swelling
	-	Red blood cells pass through leaky, newly forming capillaries
	-	Few macrophages appear
24 to 48 hours	-	Breakdown of neutrophils
	-	Increased macrophages
	-	Axonal retraction balls are visible by H&E (hematoxylin and eosin)

continued on next page

Table 1.4 *continued*

48 to 72 hours	- Axonal retraction balls prominent - Hemosiderin-laden macrophages - Red blood cell breakdown
3 to 6 days	- Intense neovascular proliferation - First appearance of reactive astrocytes
7 to 14 days	- Increased astrocytic response - Decrease in the amount of edema and hemorrhage - Hematoidin - Mineralization of neurons
14 to 28 days	- Increased mineralization of neurons - Coagulation necrosis
Up to 1 year	- Remaining macrophages - Glial-lined cyst

Source:

[1] Hardman, J.M. Microscopy of traumatic central nervous system injuries. In Peper, J.A., and Wecht, C.H., eds. Microscopic Diagnosis in Forensic Pathology. Springfield, Illinois: Charles, C. Thomas (1980), pp. 268–326.

[2] Oehmichen, M, and Kirchner, H. eds. The Wound Healing Process: Forensic Pathological Aspects. Lubeck: Schmidt-Romhild (1996).

HYPOXIC/ISCHEMIC INJURY AND INCREASED INTRACRANIAL PRESSURE

Figure 1.20. Hypoxic/ischemic changes with gliosis in the CA-4 region of the hippocampus. There is pyknosis and increased eosinophilia of the neurons in the CA-4 region (arrow), accompanied by an increase in reactive astrocytes (asterisk). This section was taken from an individual who died as a result of acute opiate intoxication. Repeated episodes of opiate intoxication with decreased respiratory drive may elicit this characteristic hypoxic picture.

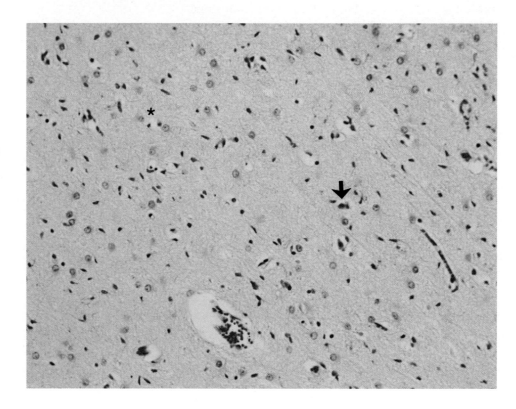

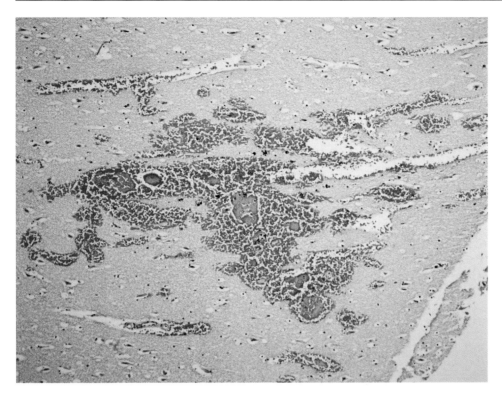

Figure 1.21. Uncal herniation. There are several petechial hemorrhages within the uncus caused by compression against the tentorium as a consequence of increased intracranial pressure.

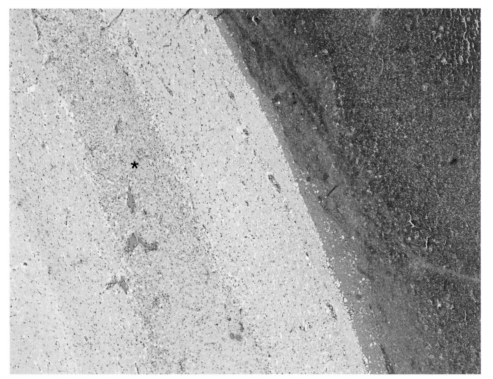

Figure 1.22. Uncal herniation. Compression of the uncus has lead to an infarct of the CA-1 region of the hippocampus (asterisk). There is a gliotic response and neovascularization with the loss of neurons. Survival was over a week.

Figure 1.23. Duret hemorrhages (intra-parenchymal hemorrhage within the pons). Duret hemorrhages are a consequence of increased intracranial pressure (ICP). As the ICP increases, the brain follows the path of least resistance and the brainstem is forced down the foramen magnum, tearing the penetrating blood vessels. There are areas of hemorrhage with intact red blood cells and areas with degenerating red blood cells (asterisk), suggesting that this process occurred over the course of a few days with episodes of re-bleeding.

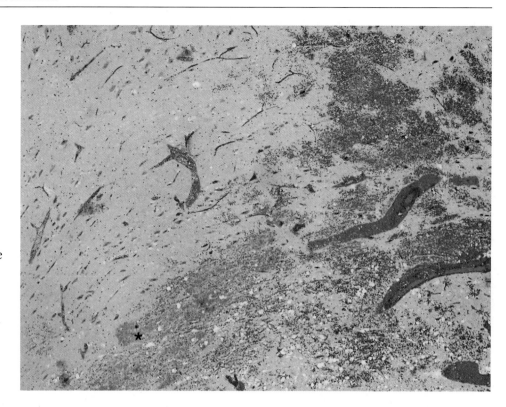

Figure 1.24. Laminar necrosis. Global hypoxia can result in infarction of the cerebral cortex that primarily affects the third and fifth layers, known as laminar necrosis. In this section there is infarction of layer III of the cerebral cortex (asterisk).

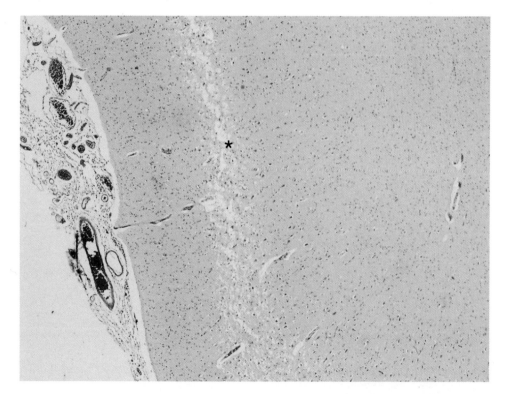

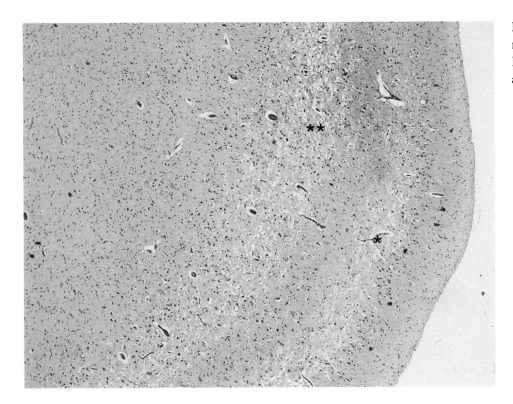

Figure 1.25. Laminar necrosis involving layers III (asterisk) and V (double asterisk).

BRAIN INCIDENTALS (NON-INJURIOUS)

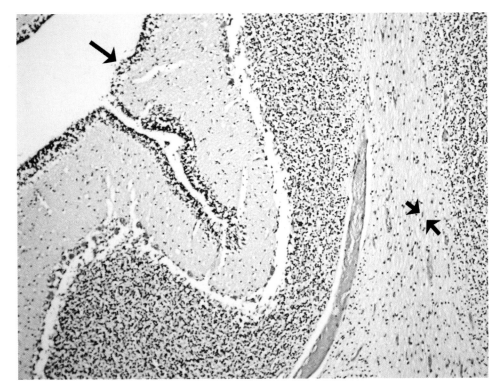

Figure 1.26A. Cerebellum with external granular layer in 6-month-old infant. The external granular layer is present and is approximately 6 cells in thickness (arrow). This layer first appears during the 9th week of gestation. It will rarely exceed 8 cells in thickness at term, though some authors suggest a maximum thickness of 6 to 7 cells. It slowly regresses to a single-cell layer by 10 months of age and may be absent by 14 months of age. However, we have seen the external granular layer at 20 months. Also present in this section are small cells with scant eosinophilic cytoplasm and round, peripherally located nuclei (double arrows) that represent myelinating glia (compare with Figure 1.26B).

Figure 1.26B. These are myelinating glia and represent a normal finding (double arrow). They should not be confused with reactive astrocytes of gliosis and can be distinguished by the round nuclei, as reactive astrocytes have a more elongated, cigar-shaped nucleus.

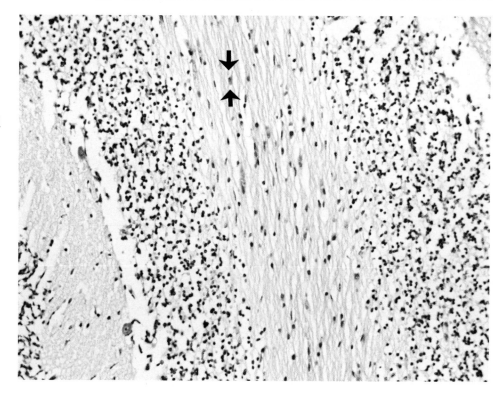

Figure 1.27. Myelinating glia. The white matter of this 3-month-old baby shows increased cellularity. Many of the cells are round with eosinophilic cytoplasm and contain round to oval nuclei (arrow). These are normal myelinating glia and do not represent a gliotic response to injury. These special glia cells will persist throughout the myelinating process and can be found in regions of age-related myelination.

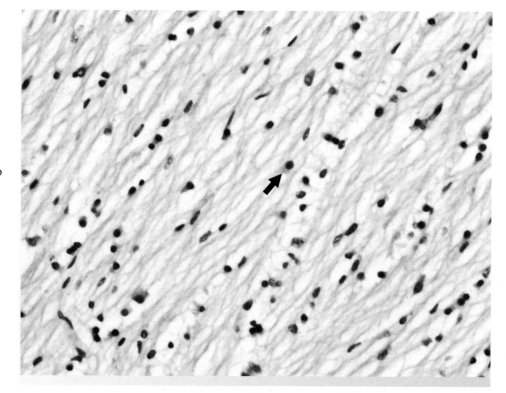

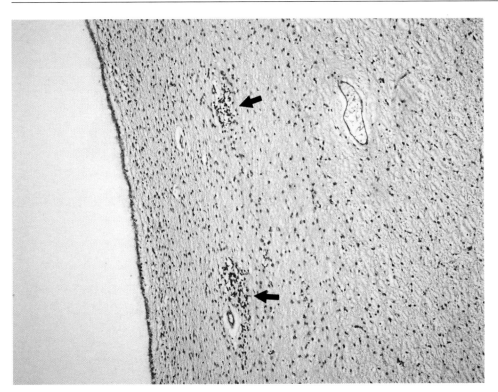

Figure 1.28. Ependymal rests. Underneath the ependyma in this section of ventricle from a 2-month-old infant are perivascular rests of ependymal cells (arrows). This is a normal finding and should not be confused with an infectious or neoplastic process.

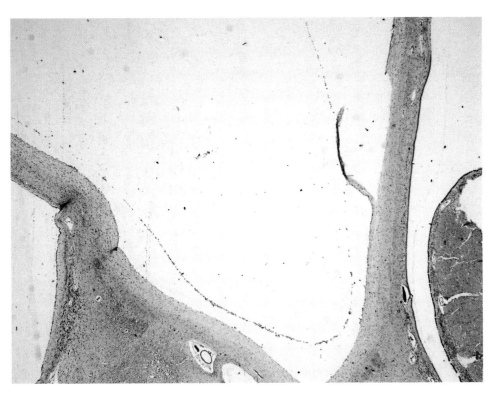

Figure 1.29. Cavum septum pellucidum. Often a normal variant of development, this represents a space between the layers of the septum pellucidum. The inner aspect is lined by a single layer of cuboidal cells with occasional cilia.

Figure 1.33. Choroid plexus. There is age-appropriate calcification of the choroid plexus (arrow).

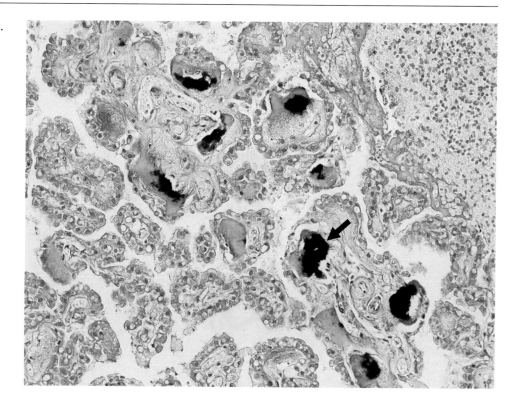

Figure 1.34. "Toothpaste" artifact of the spinal cord. Notice the inappropriate spinal cord material within the center of this section (arrowheads). This finding results from the squeezing of the spinal cord during removal. There are also areas of acute hemorrhage related to injury (arrow).

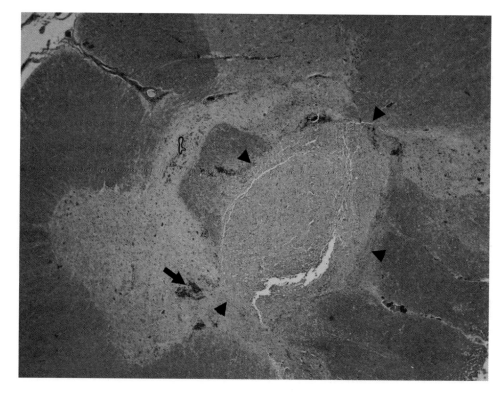

SEXUAL VIOLENCE

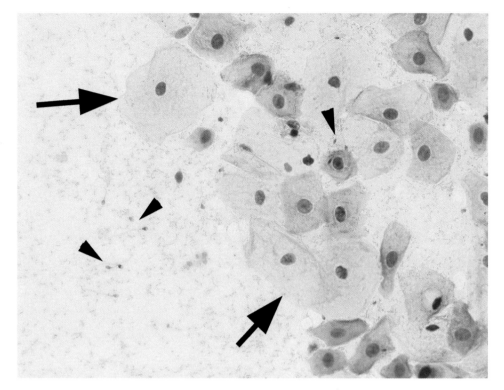

Figure 1.35. Spermatozoa from cervical swab. Smear made from a swab of the uterine cervix. Note the large squamous cells (arrows) and smaller and numerous spermatozoa (arrowheads).

Table 1.5 Evidence of sexual intercourse in living individuals.

Post-coital time period	Microscopic appearance	Enzyme histochemistry
<12 hours	- Motile sperm with tails	- Acid phosphatase positive - P30 positive
12–24 hours	- Non-motile sperm with tails	**18–24 hours**: Acid phosphatase becomes undetectable
1–5 days	Sperm heads only	**24–48 hours**: P30 becomes undetectable

Swabs of oral, vaginal, and rectal cavities should be applied to glass slides for subsequent staining by hematoxylin and eosin (H&E) and/or by Kernechtrot–Picroindigocarmine stain (Christmas Tree Stain) in order to microscopically visualize spermatozoa. For example, with Christmas Tree Stain, **sperm** tails are stained green, sperm heads are stained red. The swabs should then be permitted to air dry for subsequent use in both enzyme histochemistry (acid phosphatase) and/or semen-specific protein (p30) assay, in addition to DNA-profile analysis. Sperm can be identified in dead individuals 1–2 weeks after death. Sperm deposited on clothing or paper can be identified years later. Failure to demonstrate spermatozoa does not preclude sexual activity.
Source: DiMaio, D., and DiMaio, V.J.M. Evidence of sexual intercourse. In *Forensic Pathology: Practical Aspects of Criminal & Forensic Investigations*. Boca Raton, FL: CRC Press, 2nd edition. (2001), pp. 442–444.

SUGGESTED READING

Croft, P.R., Reichard, R.R. Microscopic examination of grossly unremarkable pediatric dura mater. *Am J Forensic Med Pathol*. 2009; **30**(1): 10–13.

2 DECOMPOSITION

INTRODUCTION

Decompositional change is the sum of the effects of autolytic and putrefactive forces on the body after death. Autolysis is caused by the cessation of metabolic processes that preserve the integrity of cells. Cells begin to disintegrate and their contents, particularly enzymes, work to dissolve surrounding tissue. Putrefaction is caused by bacteria and other organisms digesting tissue. The rate at which decomposition occurs is dependent on several variables, including body habitus, health status (including the presence of antemortem infection or diabetes), and environment. Interpretation of both external and internal autopsy observations is more challenging through the filter of decomposition. However, the added challenge should not preclude the examiner from performing an internal examination. In some cases, the gross findings may be misleading. Examples are dissolution of atheromatous plaques in coronary arteries (giving the misimpression that cardiac disease is absent) and esophageal rupture caused by decomposition-related esophagomalacia (giving the misimpression that the cause of death is a perforated viscus). In this chapter, common decompositional changes in major organs are displayed, along with pathologic processes that can still be seen histologically, despite those changes.

HEART

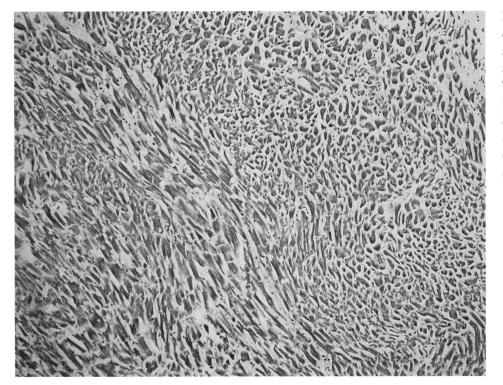

Figure 2.1. Heart. The cardiac myocytes are pale and glassy. The nuclei are mostly faded away. There is no inflammation. Interstitial fibrosis can be appreciated with trichrome stains. Atherosclerosis and calcification can also still be appreciated.

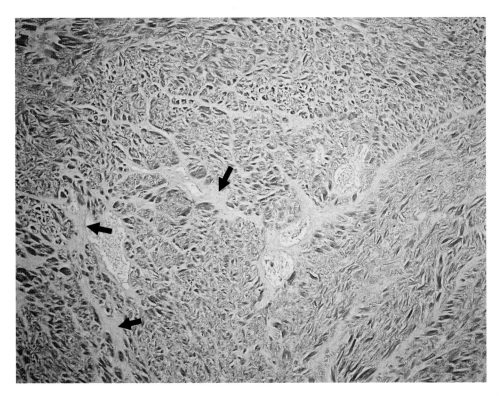

Figure 2.2. Heart. This section of left ventricle came from a completely putrefied body. The outlines of the myocardial cells are all that remain. However, areas of myocardial fibrosis are still prominent (arrows) and can be verified as interstitial fibrosis by trichrome staining.

LUNG

Figure 2.3. Lung. There is total loss of epithelium with intact alveolar septae. Residual intra-alveolar macrophages remain (arrows). Alveolar space expansion in association with "clubbing" of septal termini can still be appreciable stigmata of emphysematous changes (right side of photo).

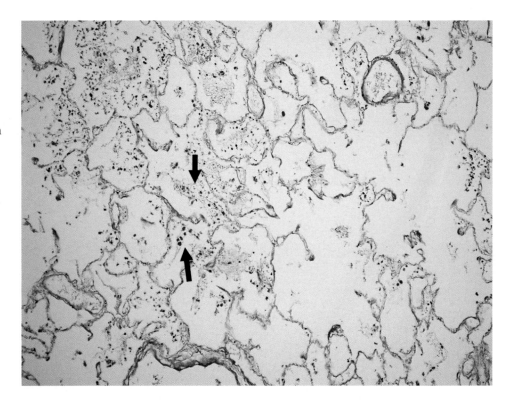

LIVER

Figure 2.4. Liver. The hepatocytes are beginning to lose their distinct cell borders and there is the complete loss of nuclei. Notice that the overall structure remains and the cells are just "ghosts."

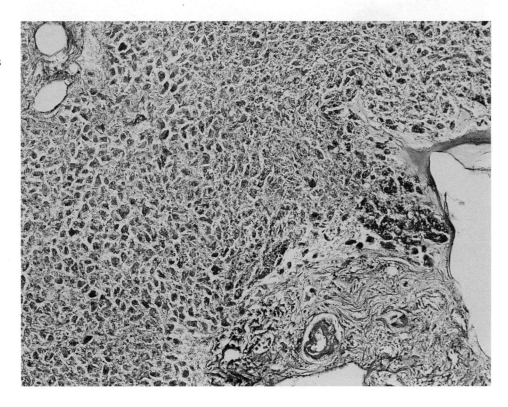

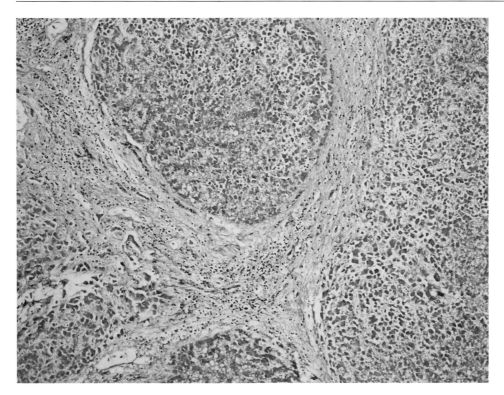

Figure 2.5. Cirrhosis. There is cirrhosis of the liver with steatosis. The hepatocytes are shrunken and demonstrate decreased eosinophilia. The nuclei are glassy-appearing and pyknotic. The cells here are "fading away" as opposed to dying in hepatic necrosis or apoptosis, where there is coincident inflammation. The fibrous bands can be appreciated with a trichrome stain. Also note that lymphocyte nuclei can fragment and become lobular in decomposition. Please take care not to confuse these with neutrophils.

KIDNEY

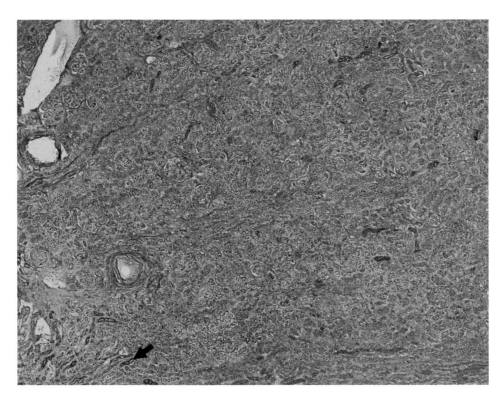

Figure 2.6A. Autolysis of the kidney. There is diffuse pallor of the renal parenchyma with loss of nuclei. The epithelium of the tubules has separated from the basement membrane. There is preservation of the collecting ducts (arrow). See Figure 2.6D to compare with acute tubular necrosis.

Figure 2.6B. A higher-power view. See Figure 2.6D to compare with autolysis.

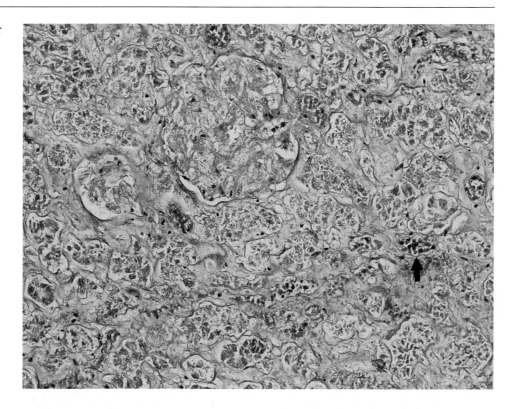

Figure 2.6C. There is loss of epithelium, while the connective tissue skeletons of the kidney remain. Some of the collecting ducts still display some shape to the epithelium but have separated from the basement membrane. An interesting aspect of this slide is the glomerulosclerosis (arrow) and the increased interstitial fibrosis (asterisk) that are still quite obvious.

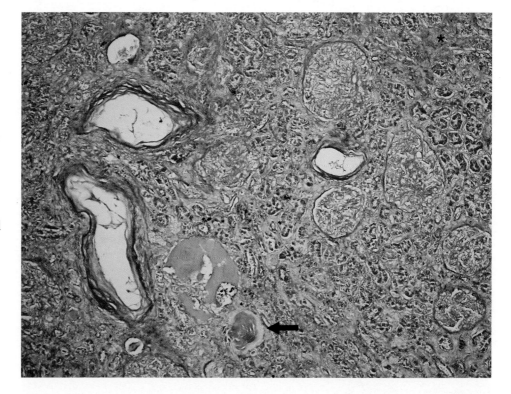

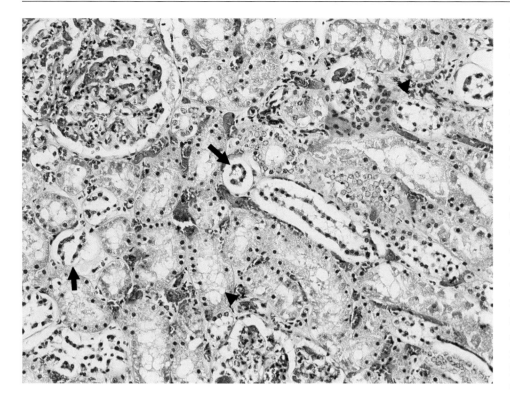

Figure 2.6D Acute tubular necrosis caused by ischemia. The proximal convoluted tubules are more susceptible to ischemia than the distal tubules. Here there is vacuolization of the cytoplasm and the epithelium has a grainy quality (arrowheads). The nuclei are still evident but are pyknotic as they begin the process of apoptosis. As the tubule epithelium separates from the basement membrane (tubulorrhexis, see arrows), it forms coils, a finding not seen in autolysis. These changes are focal, occurring in different regions of the kidney, unlike autolysis, which is a diffuse process (compare with Figure 2.6A).

PANCREAS

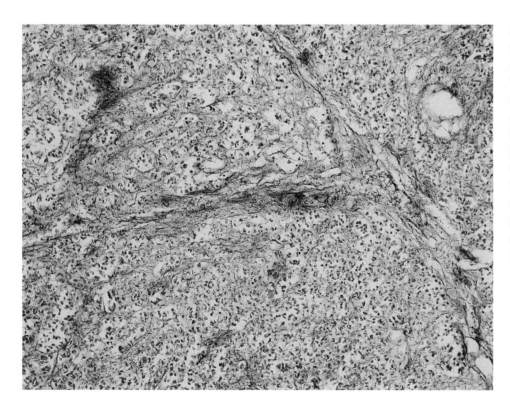

Figure 2.7. Pancreas. There is pallor of the cells with the outlines of cells remaining. There are no nuclei. This can be differentiated from acute pancreatitis by the lack of hemorrhage and inflammation. The pancreas will often become grossly hemorrhagic as it begins to autolyze. It is good to remember this so as not to over-interpret these findings in decomposed bodies.

ESOPHAGUS

Figure 2.8. Esophagus. Occasionally the esophagus will perforate as a result of decompositional changes. This causes a dark, viscous material to coat the mediastinum. The question is "did this happen at some antemortem point and is it related to the cause of death?" Notice in this section the black foreign material coating the serosa of the esophagus (asterisk). There is no acute hemorrhage and no inflammatory response that would be expected with an esophageal rupture. The epithelium is denuded and is autolyzed (arrow). The poor staining of this section is related to increased post-mortem interval.

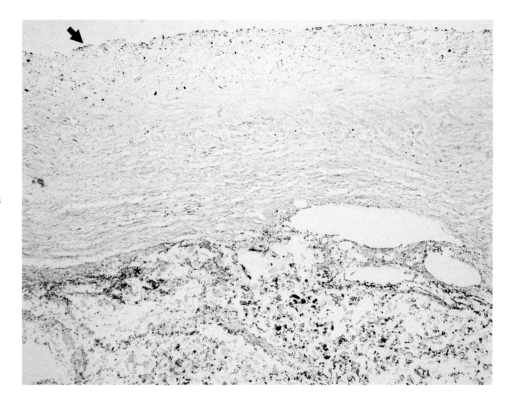

SKIN

Figure 2.9. Decomposed skin. Note the loss of tissue basophilia. Epidermal/dermal junction separation with bulla formation (arrows). Grossly decomposed skin can have the appearance of a dusky contusion. Taking a few sections of these areas will often reveal no microscopic erythrocyte extravasation.

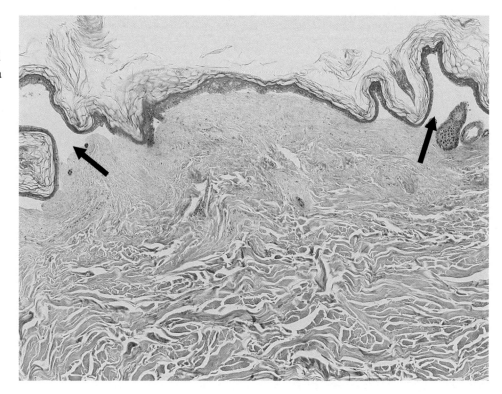

DEEP VEIN THROMBOSIS

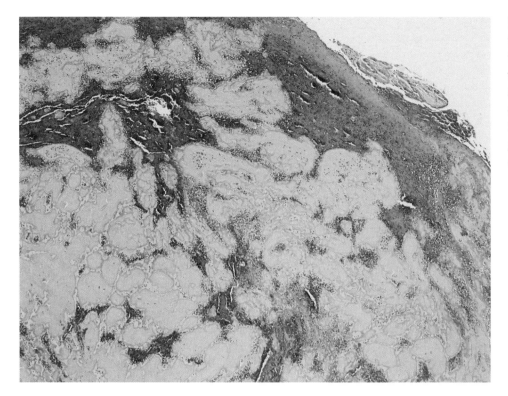

Figure 2.10. Deep vein thrombus. This section was taken from the popliteal vein of a putrefied body and demonstrates a well-organized thrombus. Valuable information can still be gained from autopsying decomposed bodies!

SUGGESTED READING

Gill, J.R., Cavalli D.P., Ely S.F. Pseudo-stab wounds: putrefactive dehiscence of remote surgical incisions masquerading as stab wounds. *J Forensic Sci.* 2009; **54**(5): 1152–4.

Kocvski, L., Duflou, J. Can renal acute tubular necrosis be differentiated from autolysis at autopsy? *J Forensic Sci.* 2009, **54**(2): 439–442.

MacAulay, L.E., Barr D.G., Strongman, D.B.. Effects of decomposition on gunshot wound characteristics: under moderate temperatures and with insect activity. *J Forensic Sci.* 2009; **54**(2): 443–446.

MacAulay, L.E., Barr D.G., Strongman, D.B. Effects of decomposition on gunshot wound characteristics: under moderate temperatures and with no insect activity. *J Forensic Sci.* 2009; **54**(2): 448–451.

3 THROMBOTIC AND EMBOLIC LESIONS

INTRODUCTION

A frequent problem in forensic histopathology is evaluating the lumina of blood vessels for thrombi or emboli. In this chapter, the histological differences between antemortem and postmortem clots are described and non-thrombotic sources of emboli are reviewed. The most common type of embolus is a thrombus. Risk factors for formation of a thrombus fall under one or more of the following categories: hemostasis, hypercoagulability, and endothelial dysfunction (the Virchow triad). Deep leg veins are the most common source for pulmonary thromboemboli, but thrombi may originate anywhere. Grossly, antemortem clots appear homogeneous, dull, and cylindrical. In situ, the thrombus is usually adherent to the vascular intima. A thromboembolus retains the shape of the *in situ* thrombus and often protrudes from the incised surface of the embolized blood vessel. Postmortem clots tend to have a layered, shiny appearance, and are flatter, assuming the shape of the collapsed vessels. In practice, the differences between the gross appearance of antemortem vs. postmortem clots, particularly with the use of anticoagulants and thrombolytics, can be subtle. In these cases, histology is very helpful in making the call. Another use for histology is in cases of clinical disseminated intravascular coagulopathy, where microscopic fibrin thrombi may be seen.

Other common types of emboli are fat or bone marrow emboli. These are commonly caused by blunt trauma, particularly with subcutaneous fat disruption and/or fractures of marrow-rich bones. It should be kept in mind that the most frequently encountered reason for this type of embolus in the pulmonary vascular system is artifact from cardiopulmonary resuscitation.

Histologic evaluation of lungs for amniotic fluid emboli is important in the investigation of peripartum death. These emboli usually occur during labor, but may be seen in cases of abortion, trauma to a gravid abdomen, amnioinfusion, and use of uterine stimulants.

THROMBOEMBOLISM

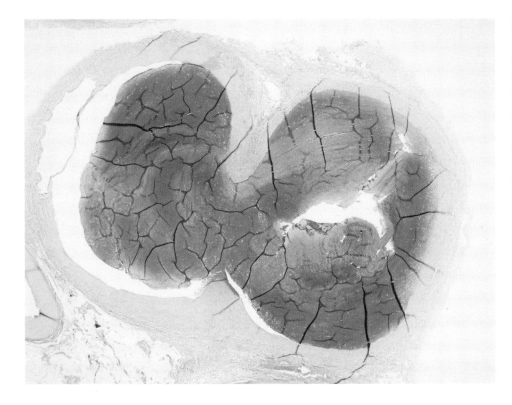

Figure 3.1A. Popliteal vein thrombosis. Note the antemortem thrombosis within the vein, which contain the so-called "lines of Zahn," representing the layer-wise, alternating deposition of erythrocytes, leukocytes and fibrin within the vessel lumen.

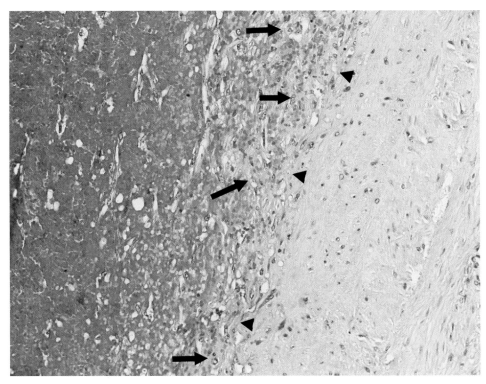

Figure 3.1B. Higher-power view reveals the interface of the clot and vein intima (arrowheads). At this interface, there is fibroblast in growth (arrows), indicating the process of organization.

Figure 3.2. Pulmonary embolism. There is an organized thromboembolism within the lumen of the pulmonary artery. Notice the layers of fibrin and chronic inflammatory cells (arrow). The vessel wall is present along the bottom of the photograph.

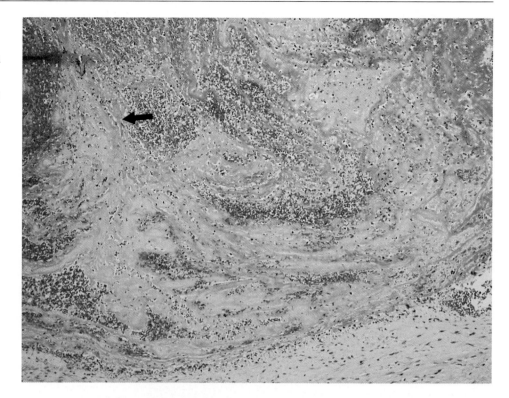

Figure 3.3. Thromboembolism. This is a section taken from a thrombus which fell out of a pulmonary artery. It is an organizing thromboembolism. It can be distinguished from a postmortem clot by the laminated pattern of leukocytes and fibrin deposition – the "Lines of Zahn" – within the clot (arrow). The periphery will become infiltrated with fibroblasts as the organization ensues with formation of siderophage aggregates.

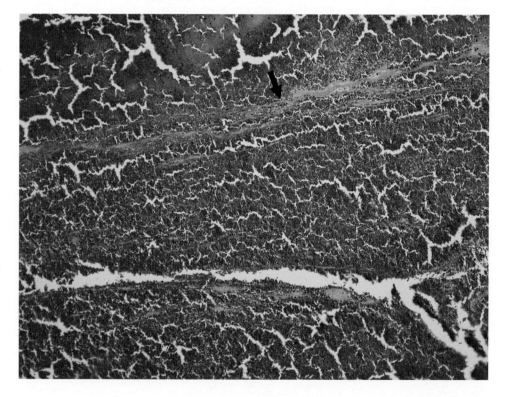

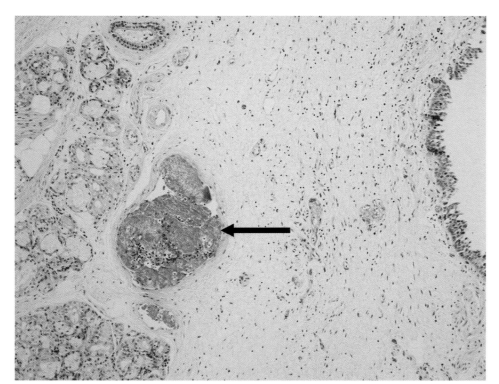

Figure 3.4A. Fibrin thrombi. Sections of larynx from a decedent with sepsis and disseminated intravascular coagulation (DIC). Note the veins containing luminal eosinophilic nodules of fibrin (arrow). These can be seen in vasculature anywhere in the body, including lungs and kidneys.

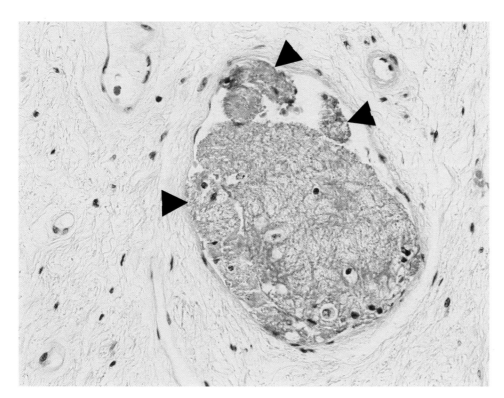

Figure 3.4B. Higher power of thrombi containing fibrin and entrapped inflammatory cells (arrowheads).

Figure 3.5A. A thrombus-associated pulmonary infarct. There is coagulative necrosis (asterisk) of the lung parenchyma with several small arteries containing organizing thromboemboli (arrow) caused by disseminated intravascular coagulation (DIC). Also present are areas of acute hemorrhage and acute inflammation (double arrows).

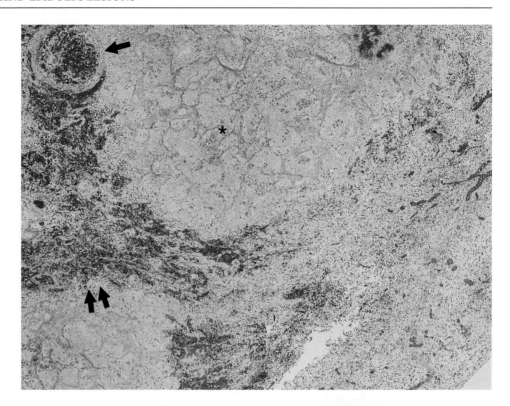

Figure 3.5B. At higher power one can see there is also early fibroblastic proliferation (arrow) and hemosiderin-laden macrophages (double arrows). The necrosis is also easily seen (asterisk).

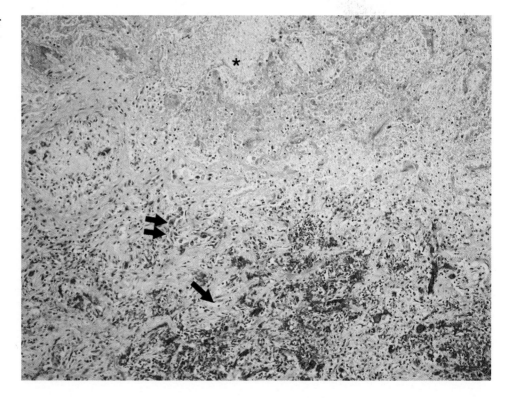

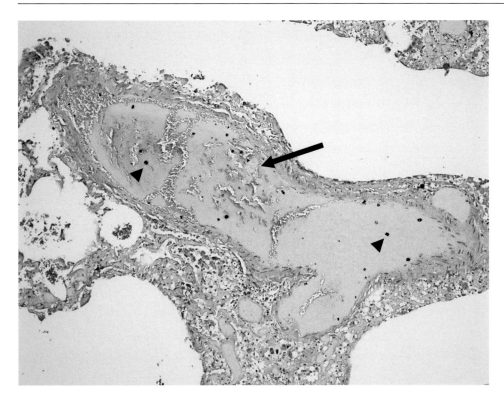

Figure 3.6A. Lung. After prolonged fixation in formalin the intravascular blood will solidify. There is loss of red blood cell cytoplasmic borders and there is cracking of the solidified blood (arrow). There is no fibrin deposition and there are no inflammatory cells. The black dots (arrowheads) represent formalin pigment.

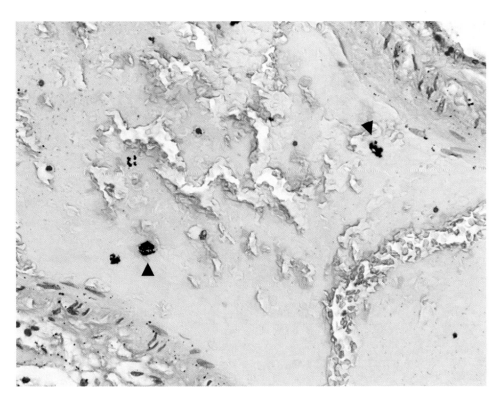

Figure 3.6B. A higher magnification. The formalin pigment is prominent.

Figure 3.7. Postmortem blood clot. This clot fell out of the pulmonary arteries during autopsy. Notice the loss of red blood cell cytoplasmic borders and the lack of fibrin or inflammation in this congealed collection of red blood cells (asterisk). The "chicken fat" appearance is caused by the gravitational separation of blood components. Within this gravitationally dependent aspect of the clot notice the fibrin, platelets, and inflammatory cells (arrow).

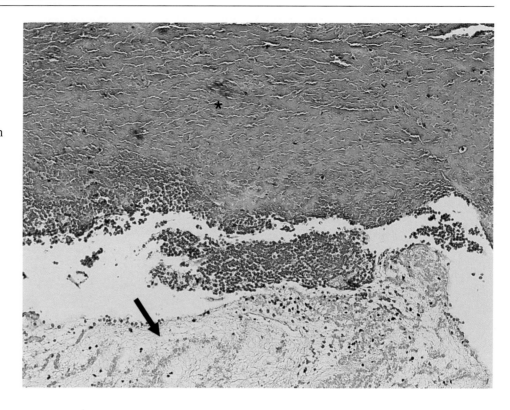

TISSUE/FOREIGN BODY EMBOLI

Fat embolism

Figure 3.8A. Fat emboli in pulmonary vasculature. Lung section with atelectasis and alveolar edema fluid. Note the empty spaces within the pulmonary vasculature (arrows).

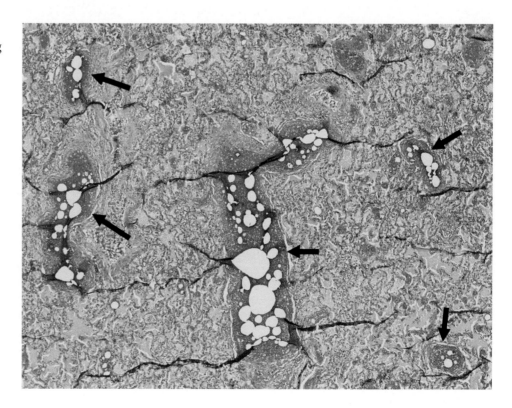

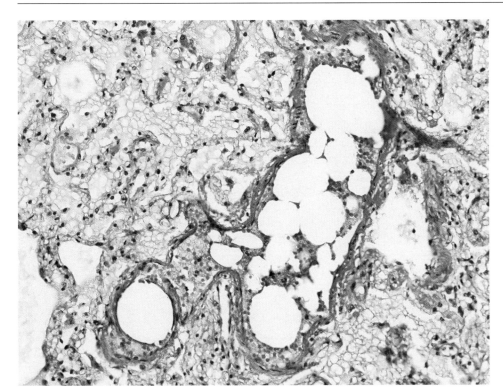

Figure 3.8B. Erythrocytes peripheralized by mature adipocytes, the cytoplasmic contents of which have been subsequently lost during tissue processing, resulting in empty space. Formalin-fixed tissues can be used for osmium tetroxide staining of lipids in fat emboli.

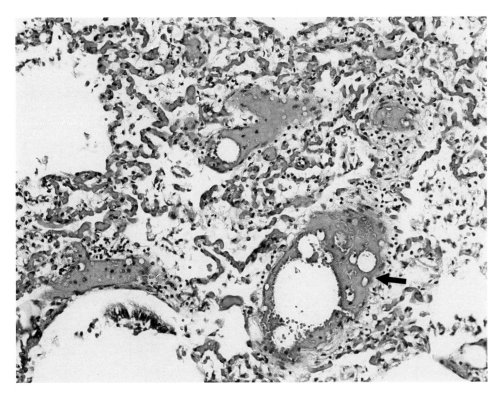

Figure 3.9. Fat Emboli. There are cleared-out spaces within the blood vessel. What you are seeing is not the fat, but a space left behind as the fat is removed by tissue processing (arrow).

Figure 3.10. Bone marrow emboli. There is bone marrow within the small artery of the lung containing adipocytes and granulocytic precursors, many of which are likely to have stainable iron (between arrows). These can occur because of trauma with release of marrow from somatic stores (i.e. rib or long bone fractures). In some cases of explosive or gunshot wounds, you may even see skeletal or cardiac muscle emboli.

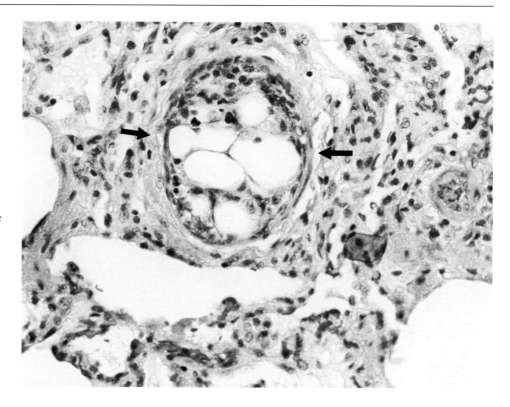

Amniotic fluid embolism

Figure 3.11. Amniotic fluid embolism. There is mucin (arrow) within a small arteriole in the lung from this mother who died shortly after childbirth.

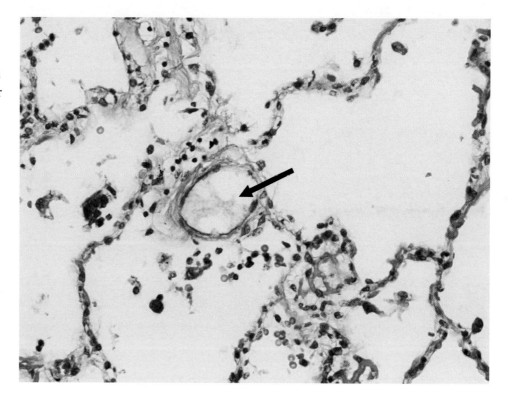

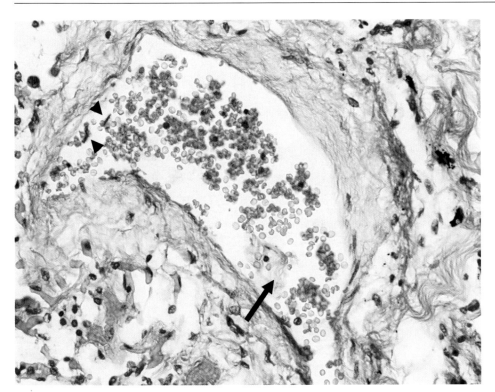

Figure 3.12. Amniotic fluid embolism. There is anucleate material within this large artery. The material contained in amniotic fluid, such as hair or keratin debris, are eosinophilic and have no nucleus (arrow). They can be easily confused with stripped-off endothelial cells from the arteries. However, the endothelial cells contain a nucleus (arrowheads).

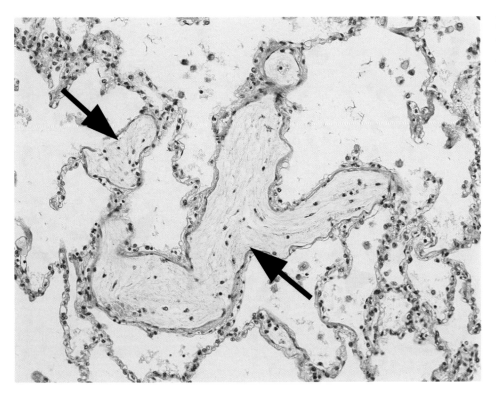

Figure 3.13A. Amniotic fluid emboli. Section of lung with intravascular mucin (arrow).

Figure 4.2B. At higher power one can see the cellular walls of plant material.

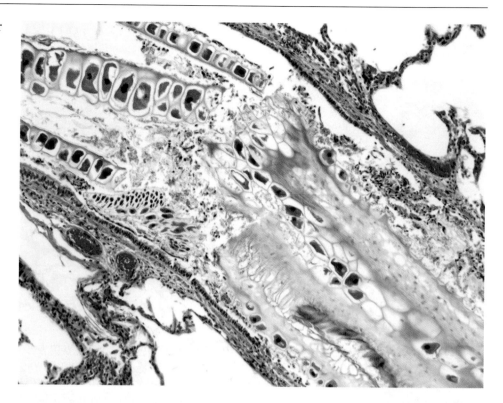

Figure 4.3A. Lung of an infant who had eaten meat approximately 24 hours before death. Several meat particles (down arrow) in alveoli can be seen surrounded by interstitial edema and mixed inflammation (right arrow). There is postmortem overgrowth of bacteria (asterisk). (Courtesy of Dr. Henry Nields, OCME, Boston, MA.)

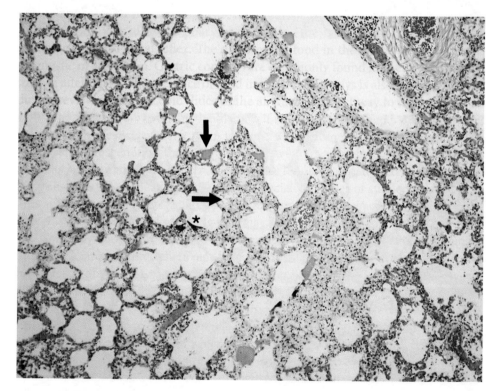

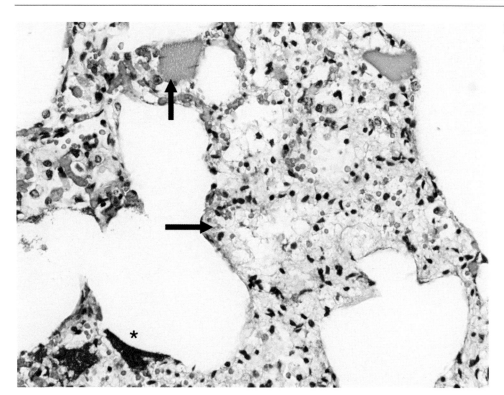

Figure 4.3B. Higher power of same.

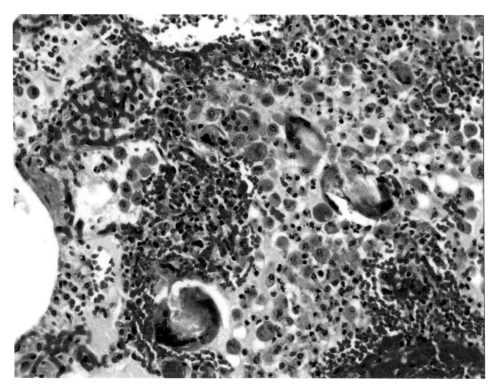

Figure 4.4A. Aspiration pneumonia. If the individual survives for a period of time a vital response develops, resulting in aspiration pneumonia. Notice the acute inflammatory response with foreign-body type giant cell formation. (Photography courtesy of Dr. Steven Cina, Ft. Lauderdale, FL.)

Figure 4.4B. Polarization of Figure 4.4A demonstrates foreign material within the giant cells.

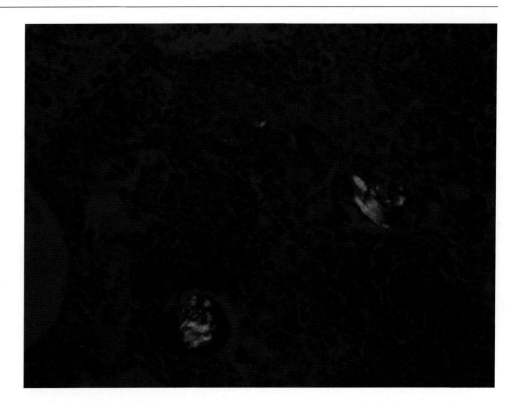

SUGGESTED READING

Kohlase C., Maxeiner H. Morphologic investigation of emphysema aquosum in the elderly. *Forensic Sci Int.* 2003; **134**: 93–98.

Pollanen M.S. The diagnostic value of the diatom test for drowning, II: Validity – Analysis of diatoms in bone marrow and drowning medium. *J Forensic Sci.* 1997; **42**: 286–290.

Pollanen M.S., Cheung C., Chaisson D.A. The diagnostic value of the diatom test for drowning, I: Utility – A retrospective analysis of 771 cases of drowning in Ontario, Canada. *J Forensic Sci.* 1997; **42**: 281–285.

INTRODUCTION

A poison is a substance taken internally or externally that impairs health or destroys life. In this chapter, some classic histologic findings in acute and chronic poisoning (including substance abuse) are presented. The determination of cause and manner of death in a poisoning requires a careful summation of circumstance, toxicology, and autopsy. Toxicology results are usually necessary, but alone are not sufficient for forming an opinion on cause and manner. Many variables, including postmortem redistribution, post-exposure survival, and overlap between therapeutic and toxic ranges, introduce uncertainty in the interpretation of postmortem drug levels. Gross and microscopic findings at autopsy can be supportive of acute and/or chronic substance abuse or may show unexpected sequelae of chronic substance abuse (e.g., infective endocarditis). Sometimes histology may be the first clue in a case of poisoning. An example of this is finding oxalate crystals in the kidneys of an otherwise unremarkable autopsy, as ethylene glycol is not detected by most toxicology laboratories in routine screening.

ETHYLENE GLYCOL POISONING (OXALATE IN KIDNEY TUBULES)

Figure 5.1. Kidney. Haematoxylin and eosin (H&E) stain of the kidney with obvious calcium oxalate crystals (arrows). Notice the necrosis of the renal parenchyma. Calcium oxalate crystals can be seen in the tubules, and in the interstitial tissue of the kidney. (Courtesy of Dr.Faryl Sandler, Boston, OCME.)

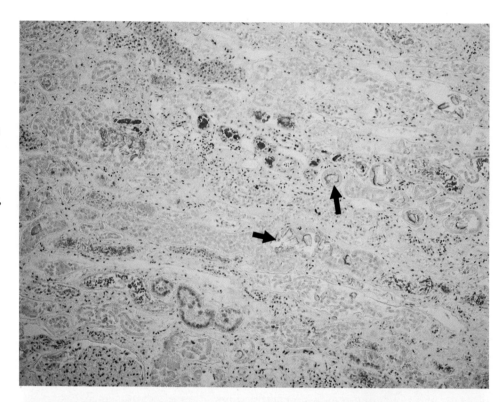

Figure 5.2. Kidney. Calcium oxalate crystals with birefringence.

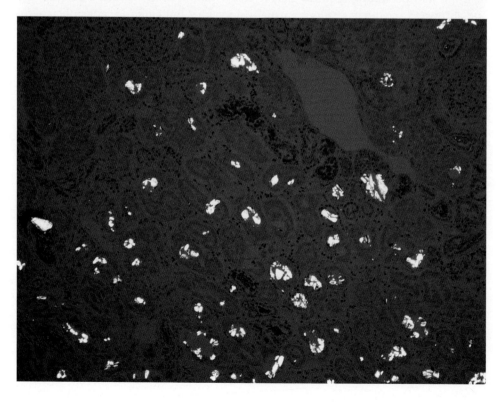

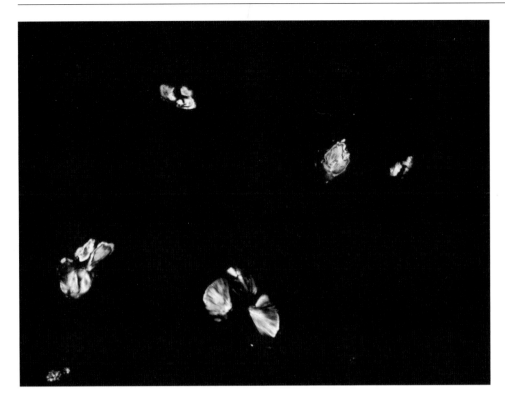

Figure 5.3. Kidney. Higher-power view of calcium oxalate crystals. Note the "fan-shaped" appearance.

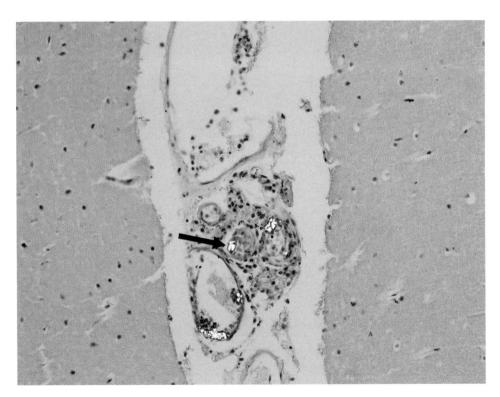

Figure 5.4. Brain. There are also calcium oxalate crystals (arrow) in the leptomeningeal arteries.

ACID INGESTION

Figure 5.5A. Ingestion of acid. Stomach with mucosa denudation, acute hemorrhage, and necrosis of the muscularis propria. Note the tinctoral change of the erythrocytes.

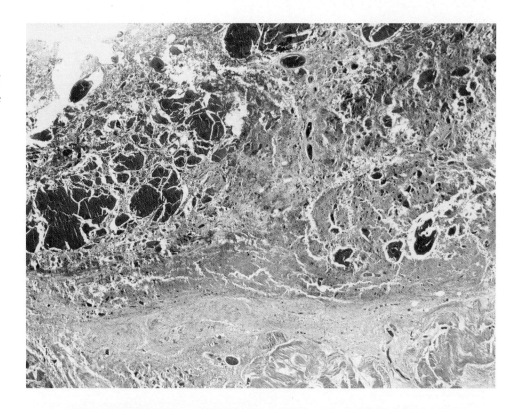

Figure 5.5B. Ingestion of acid. Esophagus with vascular congestion and submucosal necrosis.

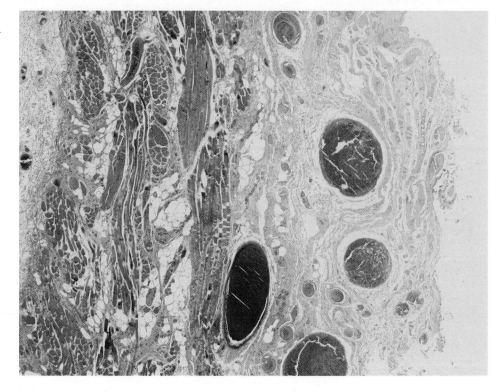

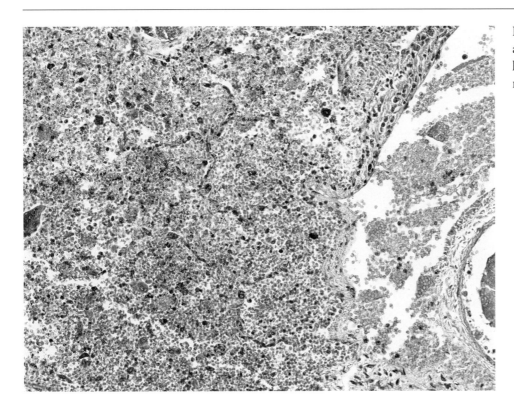

Figure 5.5C. Ingestion of acid. Lung with florid alveolar hemorrhage and septal necrosis.

CHRONIC INJECTION SEQUELAE

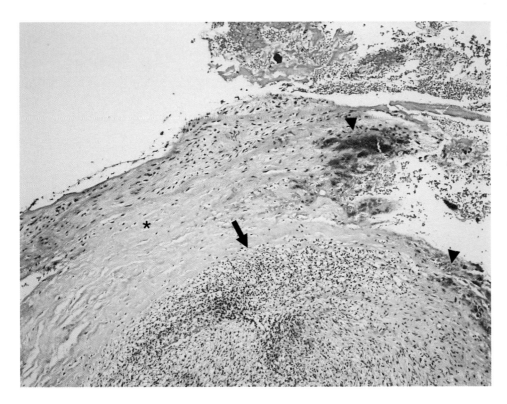

Figure 5.6A. Acute bacterial endocarditis involving the aortic valve. There is an extensive acute inflammatory infiltrate (arrow) destroying the aortic valve (asterisk). Notice the bacterial organisms also present in the valve (arrowheads).

0

Figure 5.6B. A lower-power view to illustrate the extent of involvement.

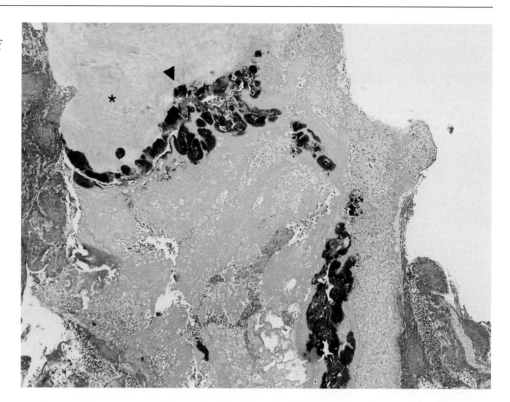

Figure 5.7A. Acute bacterial endocarditis of the aortic valve with extension into the left ventricle as a complication of intravenous drug abuse. There is destruction of the aortic valve (arrow) with an acute inflammatory infiltrate and fibrin deposition. The neutrophils extend from the valve to the myocardium (asterisk). Bacterial elements can be seen as purple smudges near the bottom of the photograph (double asterisk). (Photograph courtesy of Dr. Faryl Sandler, Boston OCME.)

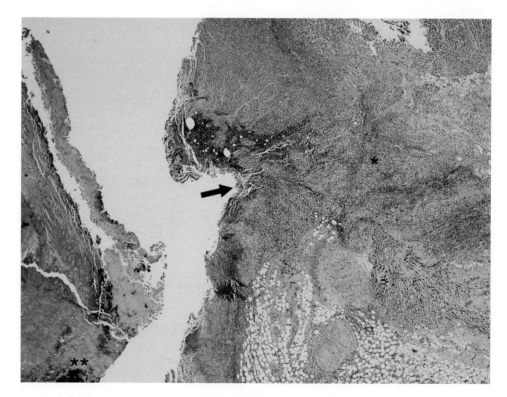

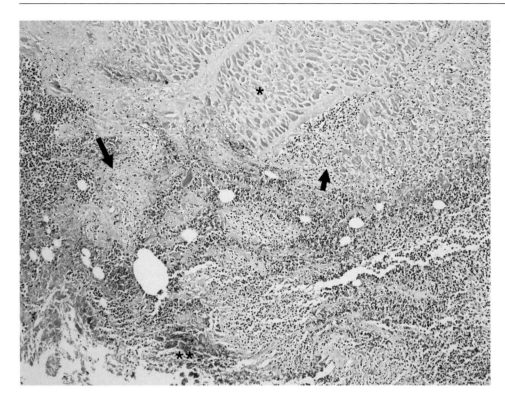

Figure 5.7B. At higher magnification one can see destruction of the aortic valve (long arrow) and multiple foci of cardiac myocyte destruction (arrow), and necrosis (asterisk) as the process invades into the heart. Bacterial elements can be seen near the bottom of the micrograph (double asterisk).

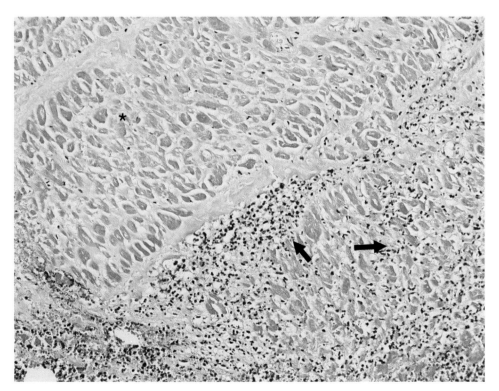

Figure 5.7C. At higher magnification one can also see the destruction of the myocytes (arrow) and a region of necrosis (asterisk) as the necroinflammatory process invades into the heart.

Figure 5.8A. Acute bacterial endocarditis. There is complete destruction of the valve (asterisk) by bacteria (arrows). There are focal regions of acute hemorrhage in conjunction with bacterial elements (double asterisk).

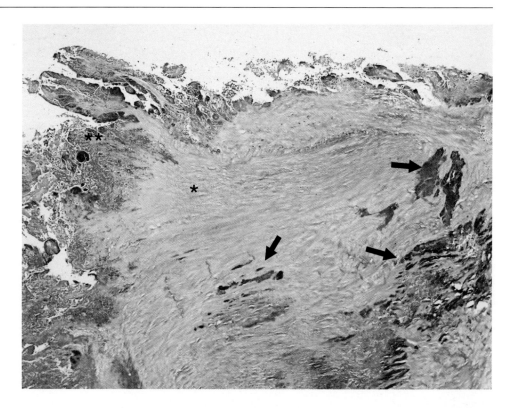

Figure 5.8B. A higher magnification of the endocarditis.

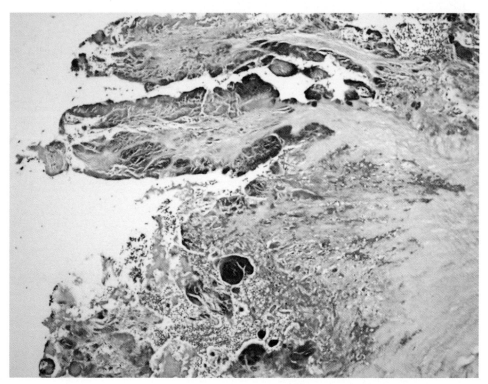

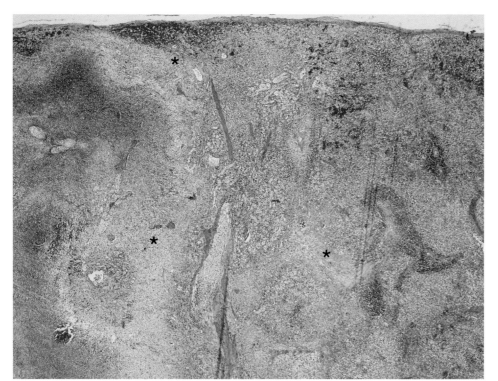

Figure 5.9A. Splenic infarct. There is an acute infarct of the spleen (areas marked by asterisks). Notice the focal nature of the degenerating lesion with preserved surrounding spleen. In autolysis the entire spleen would be pale.

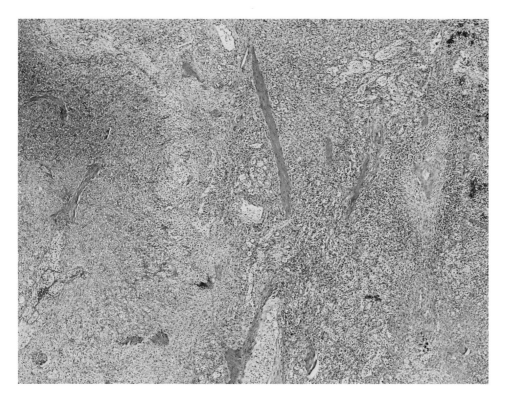

Figure 5.9B. A higher magnification of the infarct.

Figure 5.10A. Brain abscess. There is a pocket of acute inflammation (arrow) within the cerebral cortex (asterisk).

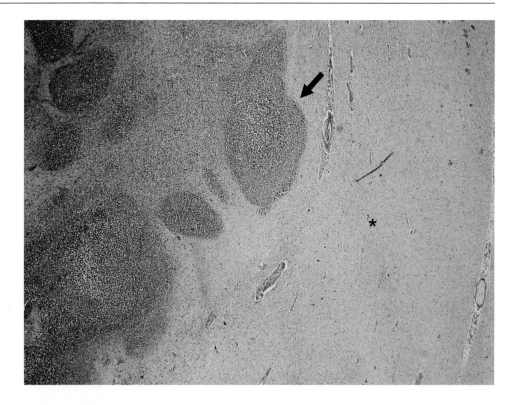

Figure 5.10B. There is acute inflammation within the cortex, surrounding balls of bacterial elements (arrowheads).

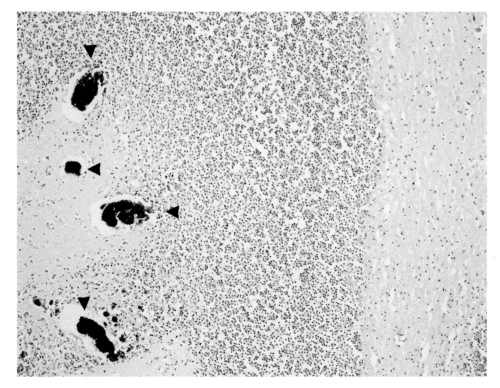

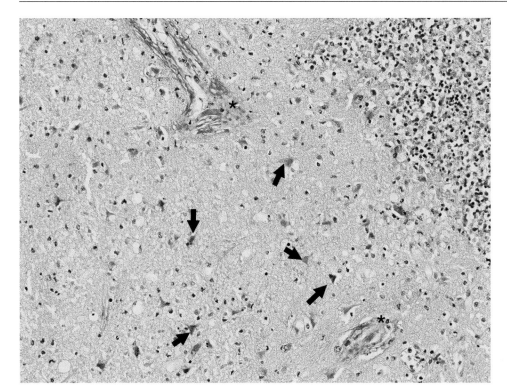

Figure 5.10C. Surrounding the abscess are pyknotic and pale neurons (arrows) and medium-sized arteries with fibrinoid necrosis (asterisk).

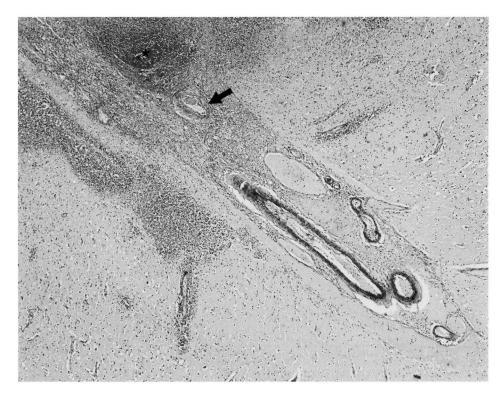

Figure 5.10D. Also present are focal regions of acute hemorrhage (asterisk) and large leptomeningeal arteries with fibrinoid necrosis (arrow).

Figure 5.11. Acute myocarditis. There is an acute inflammatory infiltrate surrounding a ball of bacteria (arrow) in the heart of an intravenous drug abuser.

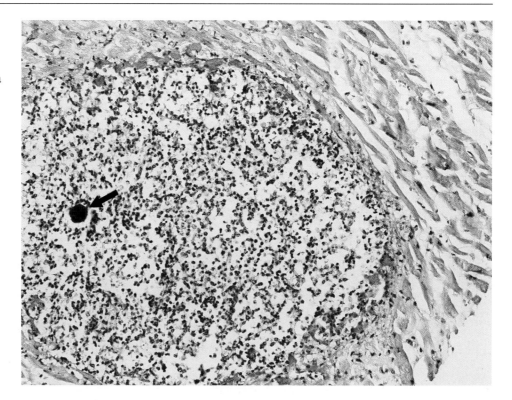

Figure 5.12. Chronic hepatitis. So-called "hepatic triaditis." There is periportal inflammation affecting the portal triad. The bile duct (long arrow), hepatic artery (short arrow) and portal vein (asterisk) are all affected. This can be associated with hepatitis, sclerosing cholangitis, and chronic liver disease.

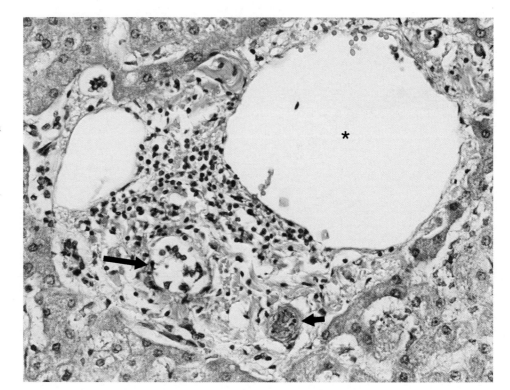

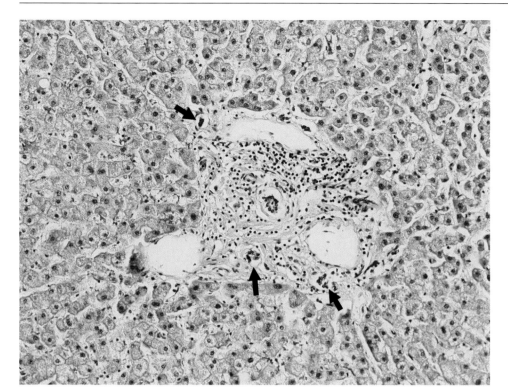

Figure 5.13. Liver. Proliferation of bile ducts, a non-specific response to injury, can be seen in this image (arrows).

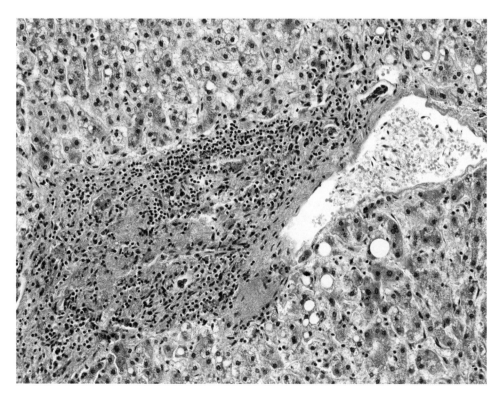

Figure 5.14A. Microscopic evidence of intravenous drug abuse. Portal area with surrounding hepatocytes and steatosis. Note the macrophages with granular cytoplasm.

Figure 5.14B. Microscopic evidence of intravenous drug abuse. Polarization reveals numerous birefringent needle-shaped particles in the macrophage cytoplasm.

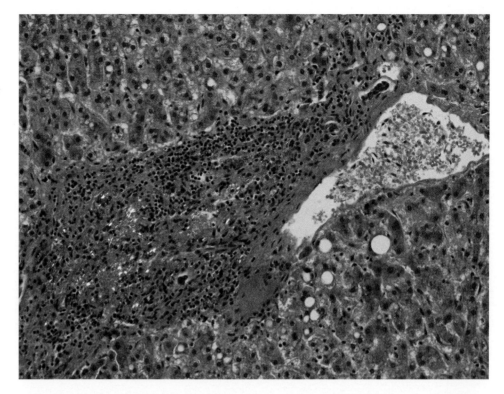

Figure 5.14C 1, 2, 3, and 4. Microscopic evidence of intravenous drug abuse. Pulmonary foreign body giant cells with cytoplasmic birefringent material.

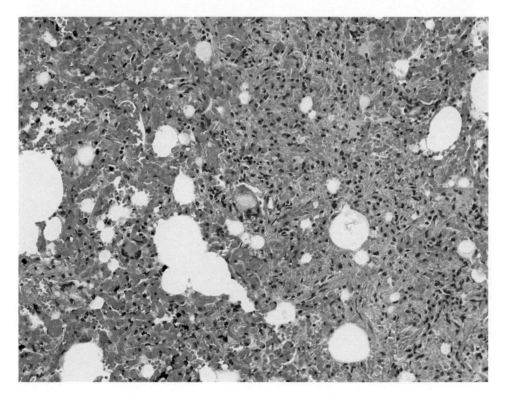

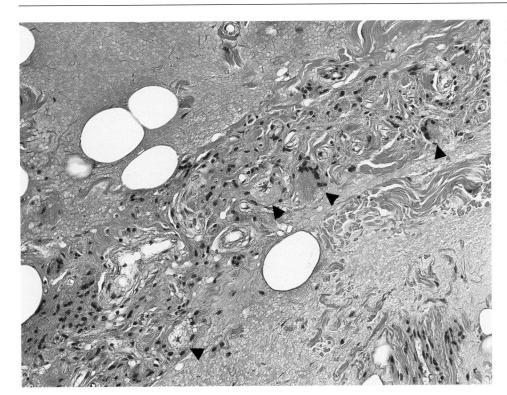

Figure 5.15B. Higher-power view of acute hemorrhage and admixed foreign body giant cells (arrowheads).

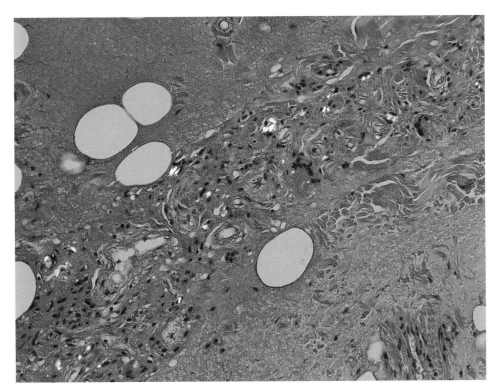

Figure 5.15C. Same area as in Figure 5.15 B. Note the numerous cytoplasmic birefringent particles.

Table 5.1 Characteristics of birefringent materials in the lungs of intravenous drug users.

Substance	Shape	Size (μm)	PAS staining
Talc	Needle-shaped	5–15	Negative
Potato starch	Maltese cross, eccentric center	20–200	Positive
Corn starch	Maltese cross, concentric	10–30	Positive
Microcrystalline cellulose	Elongated rod	25–200	Positive
Cotton fibers	Irregular	Variable	Negative

Source:
Karch, S. B. Opiates and opioids. In: *Karch's Pathology of Drug Abuse*, 4th edition. Boca Raton, FL: CRC Press (2009), p. 525.
PAS = Periodic acid-Schiff.

ETHANOL

Figure 5.16A. Cerebellar atrophy. There is increased space between folia. The folia should normally be touching one another. Notice the Purkinje cell drop out, a non-specific finding but seen commonly in chronic ethanol abusers.

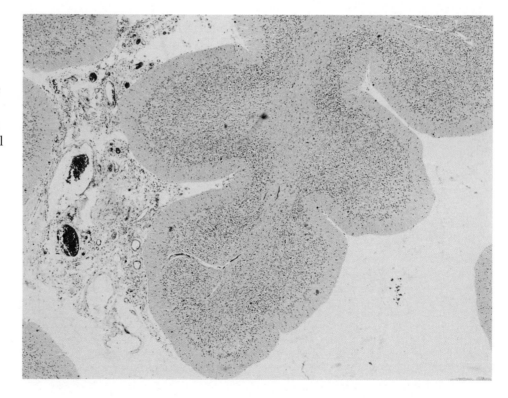

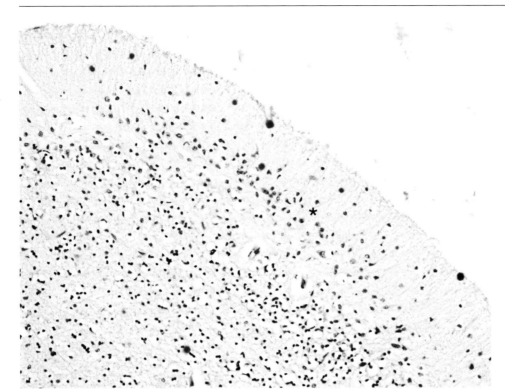

Figure 5.16B. A higher-power view demonstrates the loss of Purkinje cells that should normally be found between the molecular and granule cell layers (asterisk).

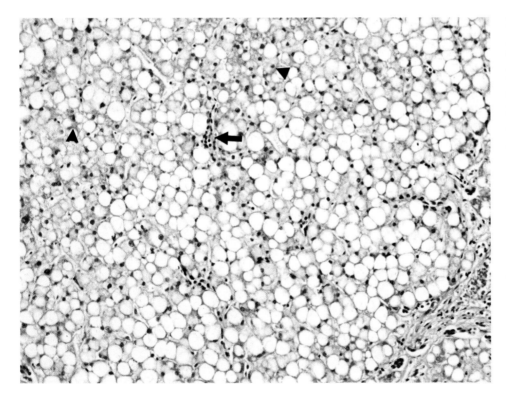

Figure 5.17A and 5.17B. Alcoholic steatohepatitis. There is steatosis of the hepatocytes giving them a clear, bubbly appearance. Increased interstitial fibrosis and chronic inflammation are prominent (arrow). Often discussed but seldom identified, Mallory hyaline is like trying to capture a photograph of Bigfoot (arrowheads). It is often subtle and represented by thickening of the cytoplasmic border. It is not specific for ethanol abuse and can be found in numerous conditions.

Figure 5.17B.

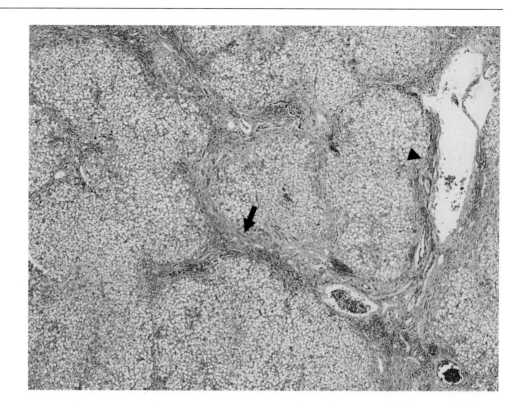

Figure 5.18A. Chronic pancreatitis. There is increased interstitial fibrosis with chronic inflammation. There is atrophy of the exocrine cells (arrowhead). Some of the ducts are dilated and contain proteinaceous debris (arrow). The islets are preserved.

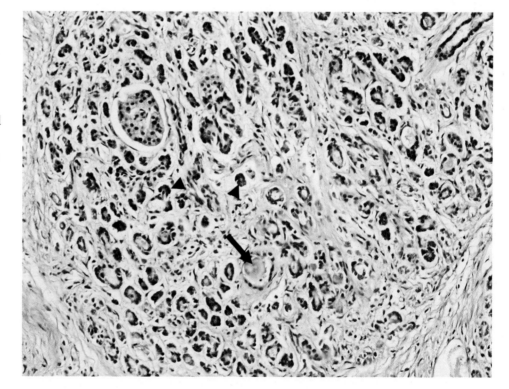

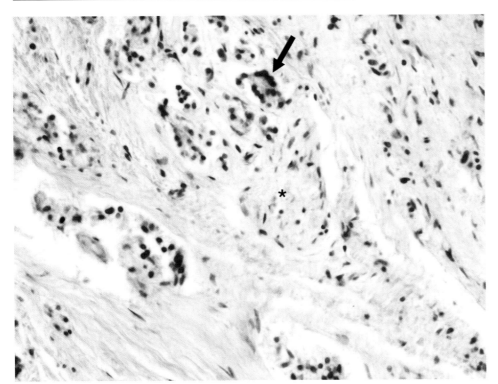

Figure 5.18B. Frequently there will be proliferation of the exocrine cells with perineural (arrow) extension in association with marked fibrosis that resembles neoplasia. The nerve is marked by an asterisk.

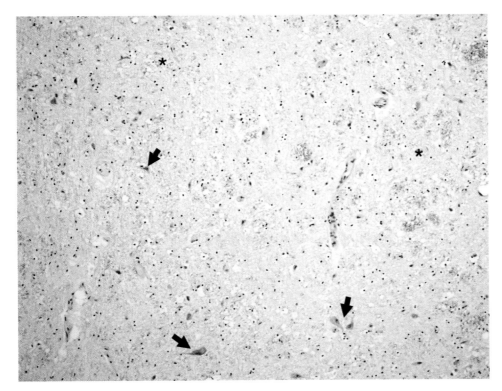

Figure 5.19. Central pontine myelinolysis. There is rarefaction and vacuolization of the white matter between the basis pontis and the tegmentum (asterisk) with preservation of neurons (arrows). The presence of neurons helps to distinguish this condition from an infarct or autolysis. This condition is associated with severe alcoholism but can be seen in other conditions such as severe hyponatremia, chronic liver disease, chronic lung disease and generally poor nutritional states.

Figure 5.20. Wernicke's encephalopathy. Multiple small capillaries with rarefaction and edema of the white matter give it a pale, bubbly appearance (asterisk). The neurons are intact (arrows), a finding that distinguishes this condition from autolysis.

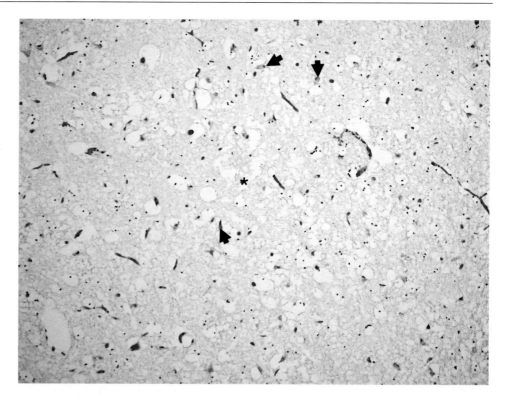

Figure 5.21A. Steatohepatitis. There is diffuse steatosis with acute inflammation (arrows) extending into the parenchyma. There is also destruction of the hepatocytes.

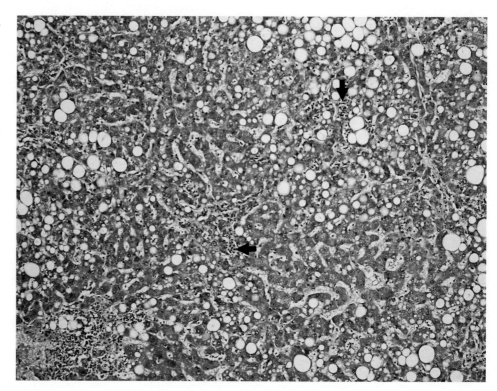

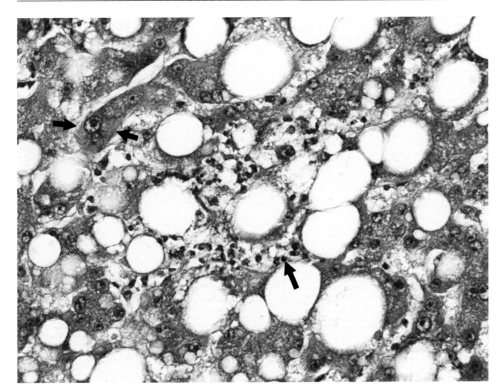

Figure 5.21B. The acute inflammation is evident at high power (arrow). Large, multinucleated hepatocytes, which develop in response to injury, are also present (between arrows).

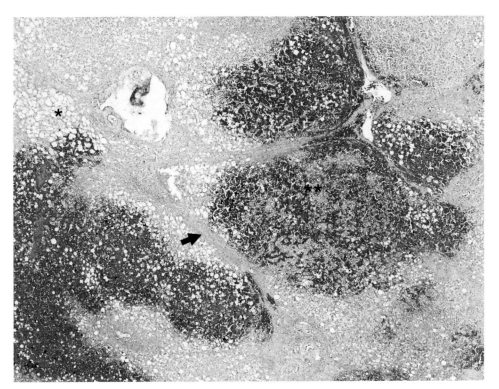

Figure 5.22A. Necrotic and cirrhotic liver. There is necrosis of the liver parenchyma (asterisk), which still demonstrates steatosis and fibrosis (arrow). There are also focal regions of acute centrolobular necrosis with hemorrhage (double asterisk) in this liver from a long-term alcoholic with end-stage liver disease.

Figure 5.22B. At higher power the necrosis and hemorrhage can be easily seen. Also note the steatosis of the dying liver. The black particles (arrow) are deposits of formalin pigment.

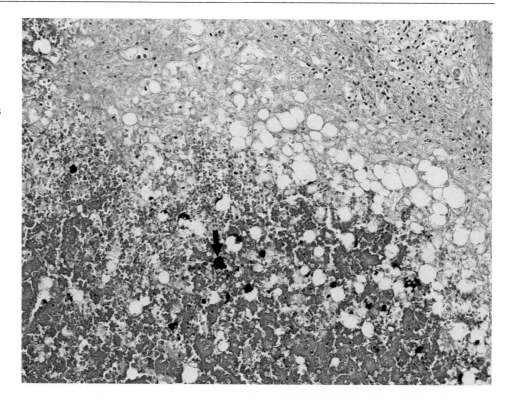

COCAINE

Figure 5.23. Cocaine-related myocardial infarct. Section of left ventricle from an individual who died of a cocaine overdose. Chronic cocaine abuse results in non-atherosclerotic coronary artery disease and multiple microinfarcts throughout the myocardium. Notice the small areas of fibrosis (arrows) surrounding penetrating blood vessels with thickened and hyalinized walls. Some authors have linked cocaine to accelerated development of atherosclerotic coronary artery disease as well.

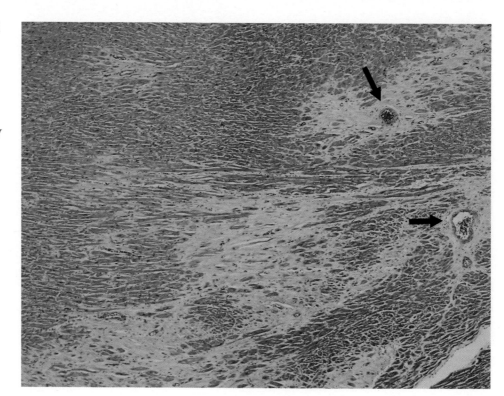

SALICYLATES

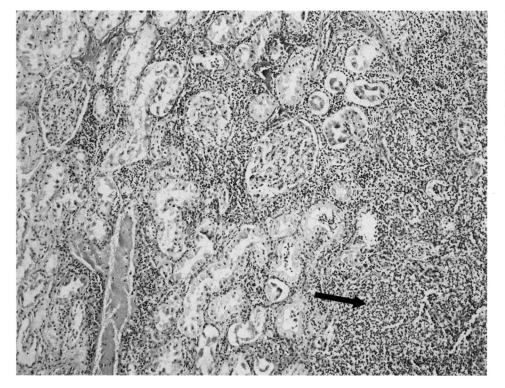

Figure 5.24A. Ibuprofen toxicity. There is acute and chronic inflammation within the interstitium (arrow). This individual died as a result of an acute ibuprofen overdose but had been misusing the medication for many months.

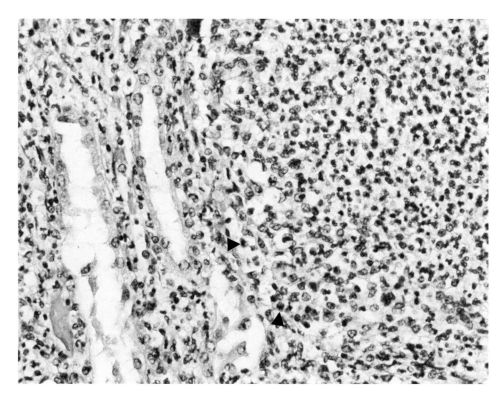

Figure 5.24B. Ibuprofen toxicity. In this high-power view of Figure 5.24A notice, in addition to the neutrophils and lymphocytes, that there are numerous eosinophils (arrowheads).

Figure 5.25A.
Acetaminophen toxicity.
Fulminant liver failure in a
person with acetaminophen
overdose. There is geographic,
centrilobular necrosis.
(Photograph courtesy of
Dr. Steven Cina,
Ft. Lauderdale, FL.)

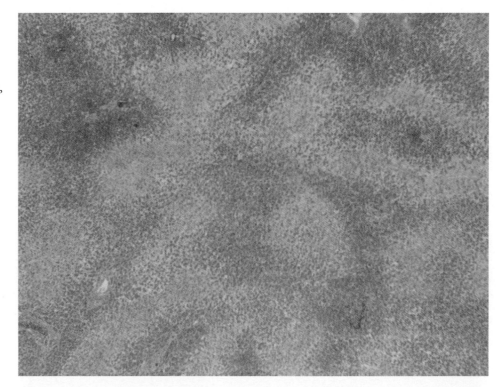

Figure 5.25B. At higher
magnification steatosis of
the hepatocytes (arrow)
surrounding the focal regions
of necrosis can be seen.
(Photograph courtesy of
Dr. Steven Cina,
Ft. Lauderdale, FL.)

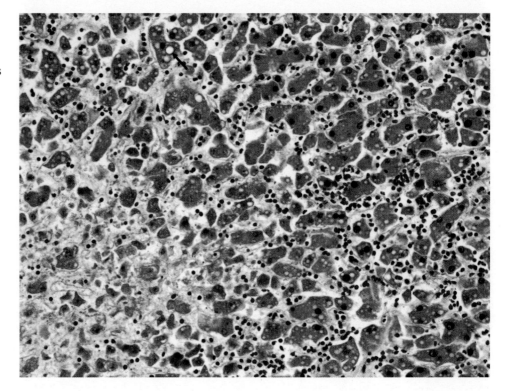

SUGGESTED READING

Darke S., Kaye S., Duflou J. Comparative cardiac pathology among deaths due to cocaine toxicity, opioid toxicity, and non-drug related deaths. *Addiction*. 2006; **101**(12): 1771–1777.

Rajab R., Stearns E., Baithun S. Autopsy pathology of cocaine users from the Eastern district of London: a retrospective cohort study. *J Clin Pathol*. 2008; **61**: 848–850.

6 INJURIES

INTRODUCTION

There are numerous issues associated with the interpretation of injuries. If the postmortem interval is short, misleading artifacts such as decomposition should not confuse the pathologist. If the individual survives long enough to be taken to the hospital there are likely to be myriad therapy-related artifacts with protean morphologies. In addition, rough handling of the body during conveyance from the scene to the office or morgue may introduce postmortem contusions, abrasions, lacerations, or even fractures. Changes in tissues caused by environmental conditions can also be confused with natural disease processes or even injuries. This is why going to the scene, or at least viewing the photographs and observing how the body interacted with the environment, can be crucial to one's interpretation of marks on a body. The discovery of soot in the airway can establish that the individual was alive and breathing at the time of a fire. Histologic sampling of a gunshot wound can determine whether a defect is likely to be an entrance or an exit wound. In this chapter there are a number of photographs that will demonstrate the typical histologic changes associated with gunshot wounds, fire, hypothermia, and electrocution.

GUNSHOT WOUNDS

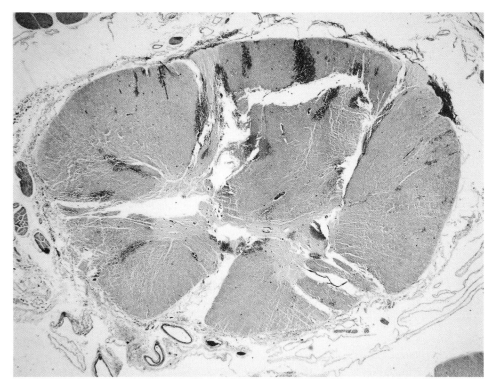

Figure 6.1. Gunshot wound of the spinal cord. There is transection of the spinal cord and acute hemorrhage. Projectiles wound not only by direct tissue destruction through crushing and laceration, but also by temporary cavitation as the projectile passes through the tissues at high velocity. In fact, a high-velocity gunshot wound to the center mass of a human being can cause hemorrhages out into the extremities and up into the neck through transmission of the so-called temporary cavity through hollow viscera and vasculature.

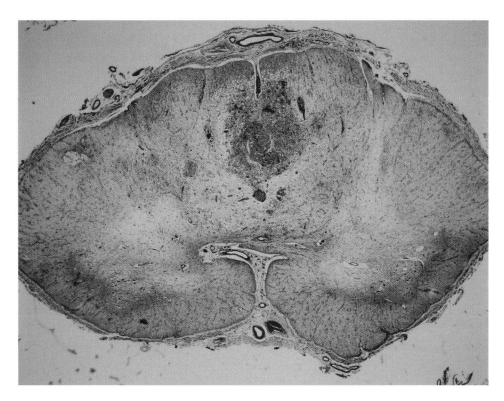

Figure 6.2. Remote gunshot wound of the spinal cord. Spinal cord years after sustaining a gunshot wound with partial transection proximal to this section. There is a paucity of neuropil.

Figure 6.3. Gunshot entrance wound. Section of skin with hyper-eosinophilic collagen, which has amorphous tinctoral staining properties caused by the heat and abrasion of the gunshot. This can be proven by the lack of uptake of trichrome stain in these areas. Admixed with the collagen fibers is brown/black granular material (arrows) driven into the tissue by both the contact-range discharge of the firearm,and contact-transfer from the bullet as it perforated the tissue.

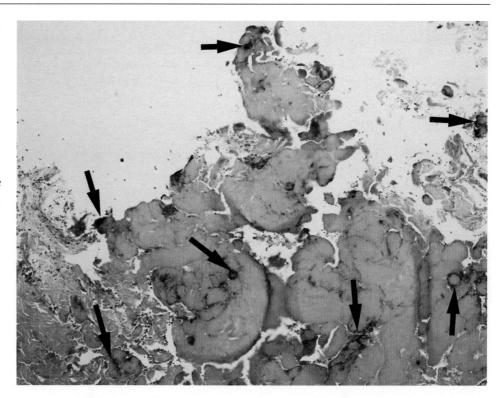

Figure 6.4. Section of decomposed skin from a contact-range entrance wound. Note the loss of nuclear basophilia caused by decomposition and the characteristic brown/black granular material (arrows).

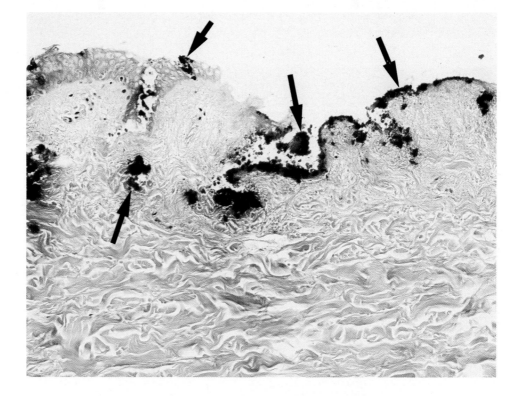

THERMAL INJURIES

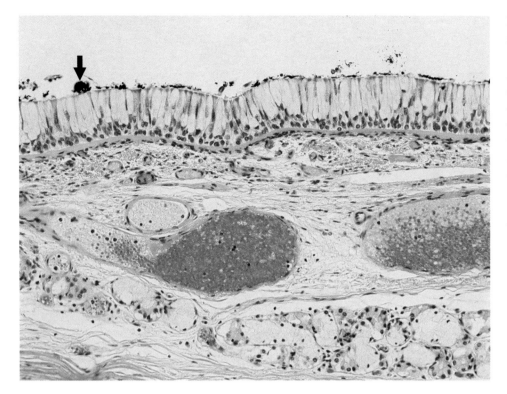

Figure 6.5. Soot inhalation in the airway. There is soot (arrow) deposited in the main bronchus. There is no coagulative necrosis of the epithelium, suggesting that the individual was alive at the time the fire started and died of inhalation rather then thermal injuries. You can see evidence of smoke inhalation and thermal injury of the bronchus together. In such circumstances both likely play a role in death. This finding should be correlated with the carbon monoxide level.

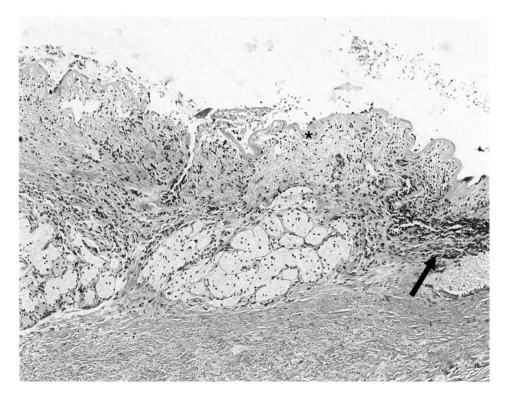

Figure 6.6. Trachea. There is coagulative necrosis of the tracheal epithelium (asterisk) with nuclear streaming (arrow). No soot is seen in this section.

Figure 6.7. Kidney. In the kidney there is congestion with loss of red blood cell cytoplasmic membranes. The cortex demonstrates coagulative necrosis of the capsule, which is condensed and eosinophilic (arrow). The renal epithelium is in the early phases of coagulative necrosis and has a "bubbly' appearance."

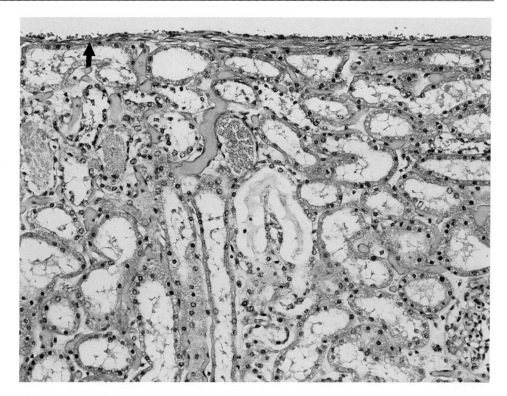

Figure 6.8. Liver. The liver shows congestion with loss of red blood cell cytoplasmic borders. The hepatocytes are well preserved but show increased eosinophilia and have a "bubbly" appearance, consistent with early coagulative necrosis.

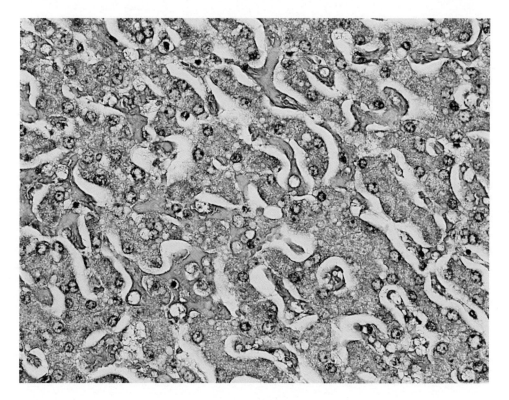

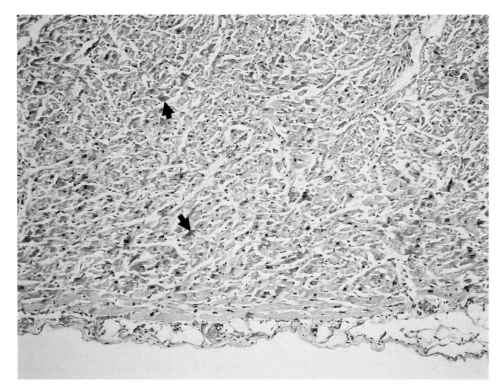

Figure 6.9A. Heart. There is coagulative necrosis of the myocardium with areas of increased eosinophilia that have a similar appearance to contraction band necrosis (arrows). However, unlike contraction bands, the increased eosinophilia is affecting the entire cardiac myocyte. There is some streaming of nuclei.

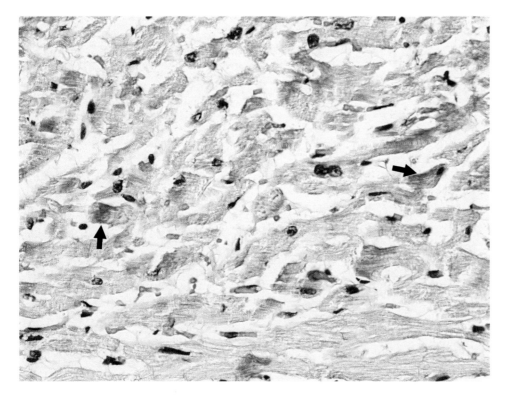

Figure 6.9B. A higher-power view.

Figure 6.10. Dura. The tinctoral properties have changed and become more eosinophillic. There is streaming of the nuclei of the cells within the dura.

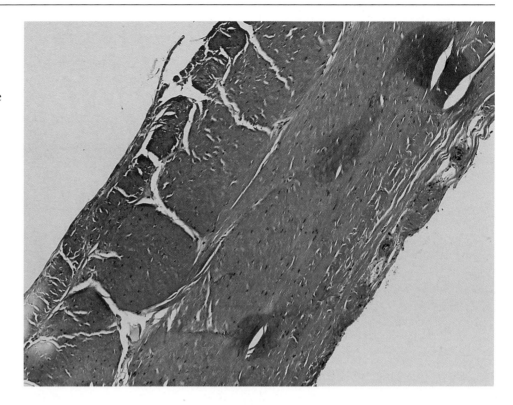

Figure 6.11. Cerebral cortex. There is necrosis of the leptomeninges, which are shrunken and show increased eosinophilia (arrow). The leptomeningeal arteries appear hyalinized, a finding that is created by heat artifact. There is artificial clearing around the cortical neurons that should not be confused with edema.

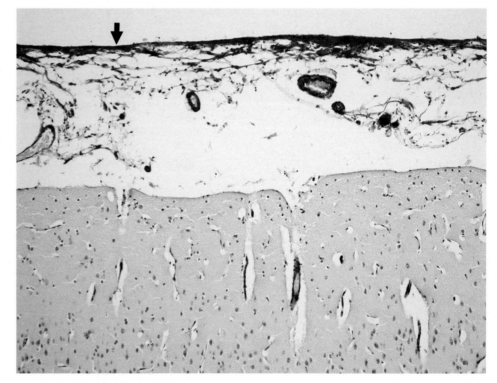

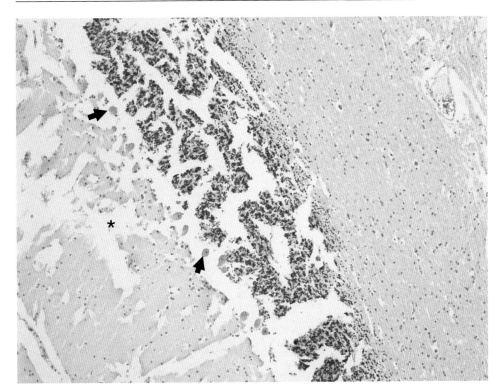

Figure 6.12A. Cerebellum. There is breakdown of the molecular layer (asterisk), which has a granular appearance. The Purkinje cells are glassy and shrunken (arrows). The granule cell layer is also fragmented.

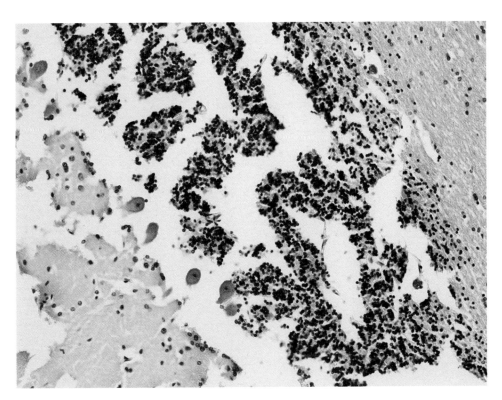

Figure 6.12B. A higher-power view.

COLD

Figure 6.13. Pancreas in hypothermia. This section of pancreas demonstrates acute hemorrhage within the fibrous connective tissue, separating islands of pancreatic endocrine cells (arrows). It is common for the pancreas to have a hemorrhage appearance at autopsy in hypothermia-related deaths. This finding can be distinguished from acute pancreatitis by the lack of inflammation and lack of necrosis of the endocrine cells. Also note that the hemorrhage is not involving the cellular components of the pancreas.

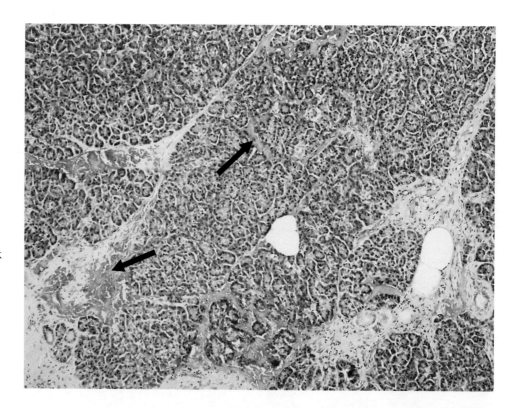

Figure 6.14. Stomach in hypothermia. Often the stomach will have a "leopard skin" gross appearance at autopsy, the so-called "Wisnewski's ulcers." However, there has been little histologic correlate with this finding, save for apical mucosal necrosis (arrow) with and without focal hemorrhage, and changes in the tinctoral properties of the oxyntic mucosa. Notice the lack of hemorrhage in this stomach section.

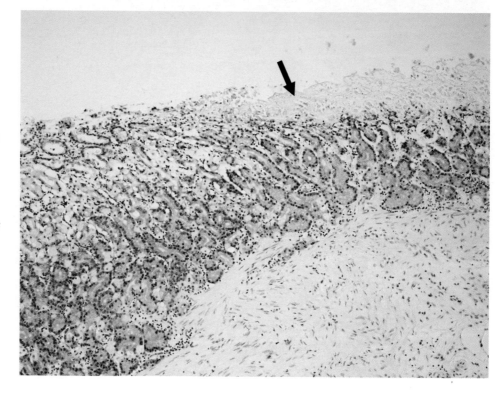

ELECTRICAL

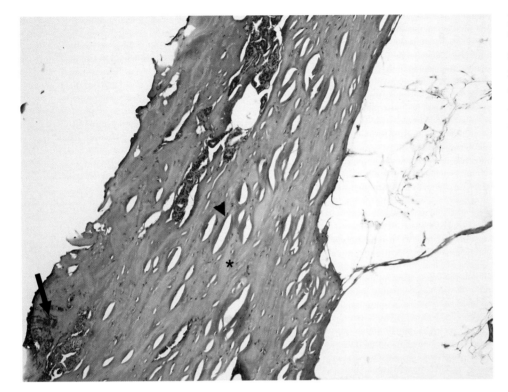

Figure 6.15. Electrocution. This section of skin demonstrates coagulative necrosis of the squamous epithelium, giving the section a glassy purple/pink appearance (asterisk). There are also large vacuoles present (arrowhead). The nuclei of the epithelium become wavy and stretched out (arrow).

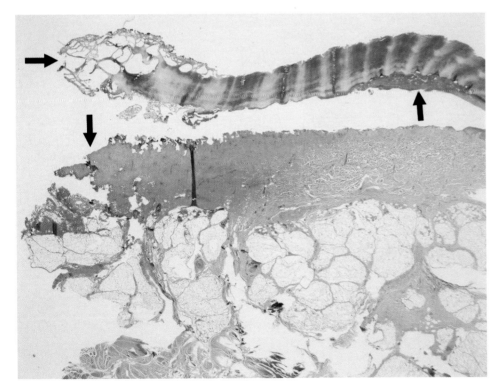

Figure 6.16. Electrocution. Acral skin section of a person who was electrocuted while working near power lines. There is separation of the epidermis from the dermis (↑) and the epidermis has microblisters, best seen in the thick stratum corneum (→). The microblisters represent channels made by escaping steam. The dermal collagen is denatured, producing homogenous, pronounced hematoxylin staining (↓). Compare it with the dermal collagen on the right side of the photo.

Figure 6.17. Electrocution. High power view of the epidermis with microblisters (arrow) and streaming of nuclei.

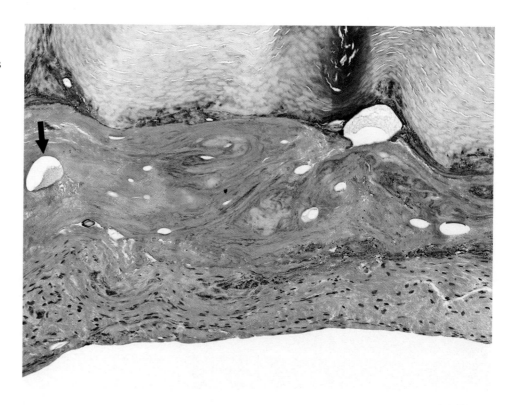

Figure 6.18. Electrocution. High power view of dermis and subcutaneous tissue with streaming of nuclei.

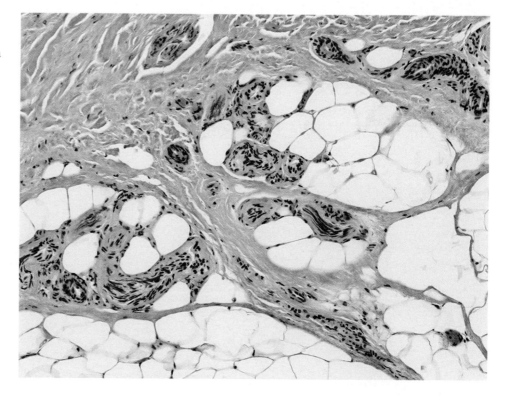

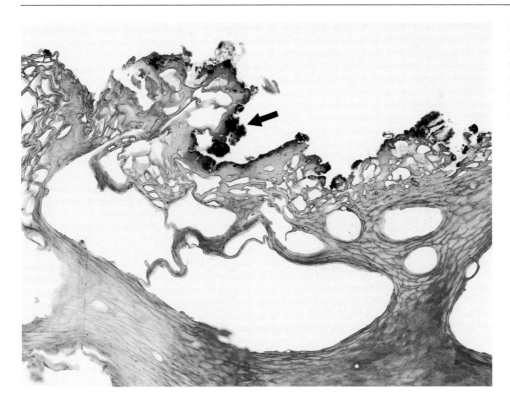

Figure 6.19. Electrocution. Microblisters in the stratum corneum with charring of the surface (arrow). Metal fragments from the point of skin contact may be seen.

SUGGESTED READING

Fineschi, V., Karch, S.B., D'Errico, S.D., *et al.* Cardiac pathology in death from electrocution. *Int J Legal Med.* 2006; **123**(2): 1437–1596.

Tsokos, M., Rothschild, M.A., Madea, B., Ribe, M., Sperhake, J.P. Histological and immunohistochemical study of Wischnewsky spots in fatal hypothermia. *Am J Forensic Med Pathol.* 2006; **27**(1): 70–74.

7   SUDDEN DEATH

INTRODUCTION

The majority of deaths investigated by forensic pathologists will be certified as natural. The use of appropriate microscopy in these cases will assist the pathologist in identifying the disease process and any other underlying medical condition that may exist. One can logically assume that any "sudden death" is most likely owing to some catastrophic cardiovascular or cerebrovascular event. Most cases of natural death will involve what is known as "sudden cardiac death." Histologic sampling of the myocardium may reveal an acute infarct or an old scar that may have resulted in dysrhythmia. Histology may also demonstrate hypertensive changes in the vasculature of the kidney or cerebrum, or may reveal stigmata of healing from ischemic injuries in the heart, such as multifocal interstitial fibrosis, in the absence of gross findings.

Occasionally the microscopy may corroborate or detect congenital diseases that may have tremendous implications for families, such as idiopathic hypertrophic subaortic stenosis from Anderson–Fabry disease. Deaths related to seizure disorders are also common in forensic practice. Often the examination sheds no light on the eliptogenic origin, but occasionally tumors are discovered or cortical dysplasias may be found. As the population ages, medical care improves and terminal diseases behave more like chronic conditions such that Human Immunodeficiency Virus-related diseases may become more commonplace and may cause the re-interpretation of natural disease states. In this chapter there are numerous photographs of the natural disease processes we commonly encounter.

CARDIOVASCULAR SYSTEM

Hypertension

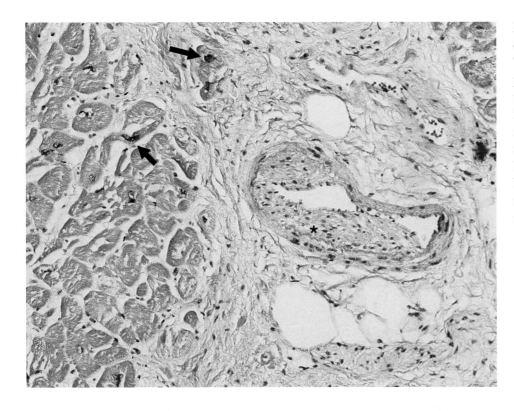

Figure 7.1. Small-vessel disease in hypertension. The subintima of this small penetrating arteriole is thickened and displays increased cellularity, reflecting the hyperplasia of subintimal cells (asterisk). Notice the enlarged, box-shaped nuclei of the surrounding cardiac myocytes (arrows).

Figure 7.2. Hypertension. The nuclei of the hypertrophic cardiac myocytes are enlarged and box-shaped (arrows).

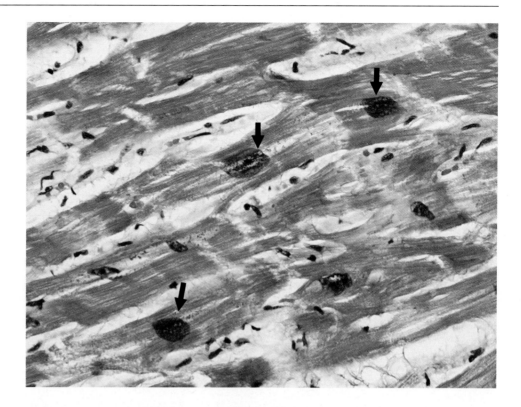

Figure 7.3A. Atheroma of pulmonary artery. There is an increase in the thickness of the intima with cholesterol deposition. The arrow marks the endothelial lining. The pulmonary circuit is low pressure and should not have atheromatosis. Therefore, the presence of pulmonary artery atheromata indicates chronic pulmonary hypertension.

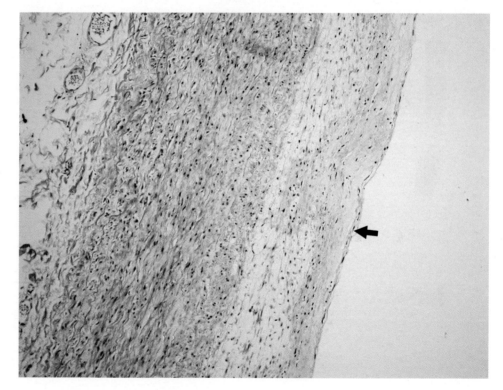

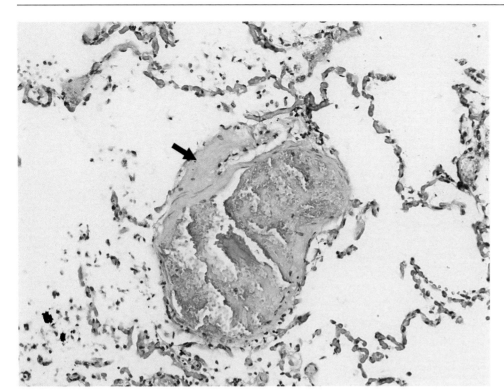

Figure 7.3B. Atheroma of pulmonary artery within the lung parenchyma (arrow). Notice how the artery is thickened, much like the changes seen in the coronary arteries in atherosclerosis.

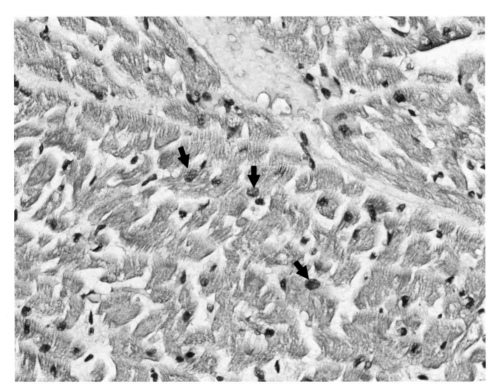

Figure 7.4. Right ventricular hypertrophy caused by pulmonary hypertension. Just as the left ventricle enlarges as a result of increased systemic blood pressure, the right ventricle increases as a consequence of increased pulmonary pressures. Notice the enlarged nuclei (arrows) of the right ventricular cardiac myocytes, which should normally be thinner and more delicate.

Figure 7.5A. Dissection of carotid artery caused by hypertension. In this low-power view there is acute hemorrhage between the intima (asterisk) and media.

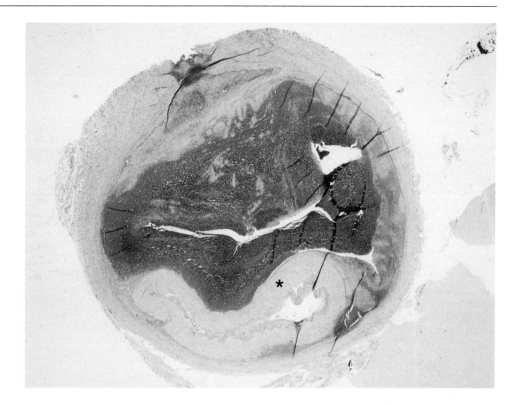

Figure 7.5B. Dissection of carotid artery. At higher magnification, an acute inflammatory infiltrate is accompanied by early invasion by lymphocytes and fibrin deposition (arrow). An asterisk marks the lumen of the artery.

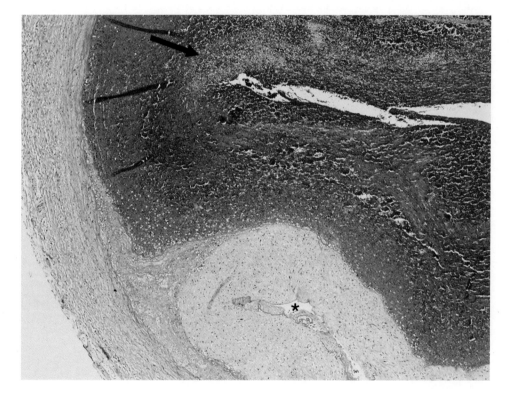

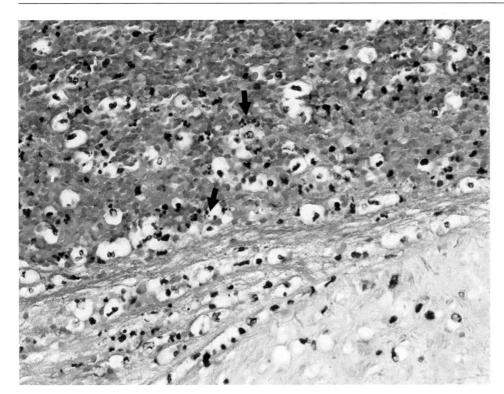

Figure 7.5C. Dissection of carotid artery. At an even higher magnification some of the neutrophils are beginning to break down producing "neutrophilic dust" (arrows). An additional finding in the section is the loss of red blood cell cytoplasmic borders in some regions. Red blood cells begin to dissolve after 3 to 5 days. This finding suggests the dissection is approximately 5 days old.

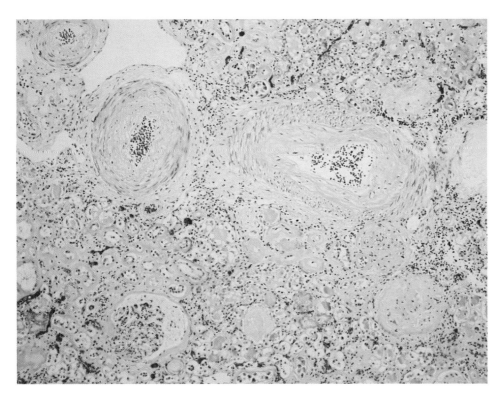

Figure 7.6A. Renal hypertensive changes. Section of kidney with numerous arteries and arterioles demonstrating subintimal hyperplasia.

Figure 7.6B. Higher-power view revealing subintimal hyperplasia and hypertrophy of the vascular media (arrow), in addition to small vessels with eosinophilic amorphous material deposition in the media, manifesting "fibrinoid necrosis" (arrowheads).

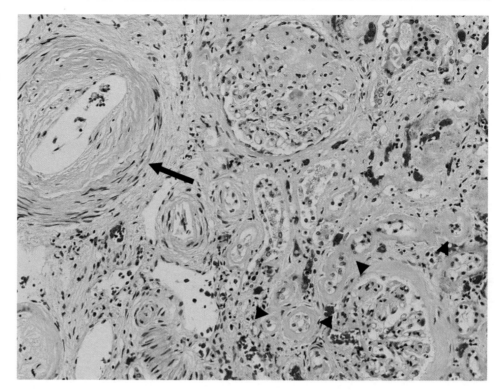

Myocardial infarction

Table 7.1 Temporal alterations in myocardial infarctions.

Time	Gross	Microscopic
30 min–4 hours	Nothing	No alteration to myocyte waviness
4–12 hours	Myocardial mottling	Contraction band myonecrosis (a.k.a. coagulative myocytolysis) begins. Reperfusion can cause focal interstitial hemorrhage
12–24 hours	Myocardial mottling	Contraction band myonecrosis admixed with myocyte coagulative necrosis (i.e., myocyte hyper-eosinophilia, loss of nuclei, loss of cytosolic detail) and neutrophillic infiltration
1–3 days	Yellow-tan infarct with hyperemic border	Continued myocyte coagulative necrosis with established neutrophillic infiltrate in the interstitium
3–7 days	Yellow–tan infarct with hyperemic border	Neutrophil and macrophage infiltration with disintegration of myocytes
7–10 days	Yellow–tan infarct with hyperemic border	Phagocytosis of dead myocytes by macrophages with development of loose granulation tissue

Time	Gross	Microscopic
10–14 days	Soft tan–white center with hyperemic border	Granulation tissue with angiogenesis and early collagenous replacement
2 weeks–2 months	Soft tan–white scar	Collagen deposition and geographic acellular areas
> 2 months	Firm tan–white scar	Dense collagenization

Source:

[1] Baroldi, G. Myocardial cell death, including ischemic heart disease and its complications. In: Silver, M.D., Gottlieb, A.I., Schoen, F.J. eds., Cardiovascular Pathology, 3rd edition. Churchhill Livingstone (2001), pp. 198–255.

[2] Schoen, F.J. The Heart. In: Kumar, V., Abbas, A.K., and Fausto, N. eds., Robbins and Cotran: Pathologic Basis of Disease, 7th edition. Saunders (2004), pp. 555–618.

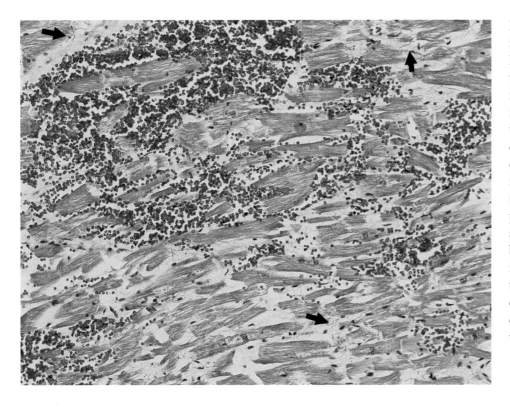

Figure 7.7. Acute myocardial infarct. There is acute hemorrhage present within the interstitium. An inflammatory response is not yet present. Also note the edema that is creating clear spaces between the cardiac myocytes within the infarct. Bacterial overgrowth (arrows) indicates a longer postmortem interval; this should not be confused with a bacterial myocarditis, as there is no inflammatory response to the bacteria. Several of the cardiac myocytes contain enlarged nuclei, consistent with hypertensive changes.

Figure 7.8A. Early myocardial infarct of the left ventricle. There are wavy fibers present along with early coagulative necrosis manifested by pallor of the cardiac myocytes and loss of nuclei. Some of the wavy fibers demonstrate increased eosinophilia, thinning and loss of striations. Also present are several contraction bands (arrows). Notice there is no inflammatory infiltrate, suggesting this lesion is less than 24 hours old. These histologic changes may also accompany carbon monoxide poisoning, catecholamine affect, and drowning.

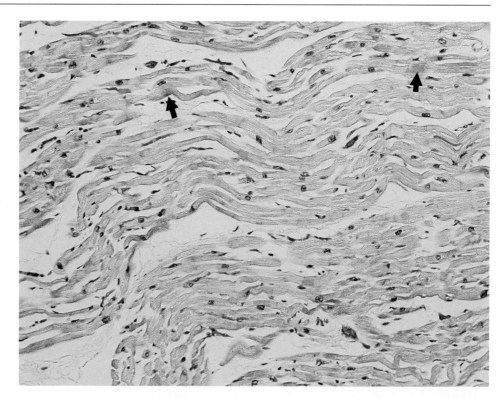

Figure 7.8B. A higher-power view demonstrates numerous foci of contraction band necrosis (arrows).

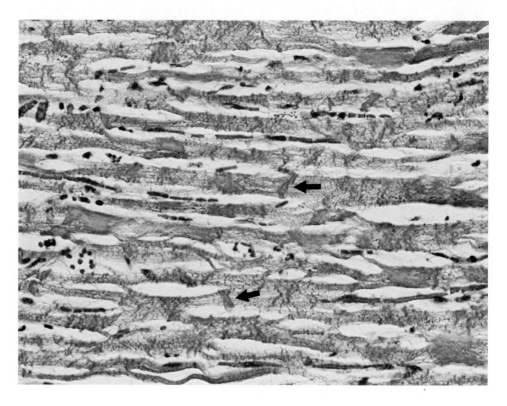

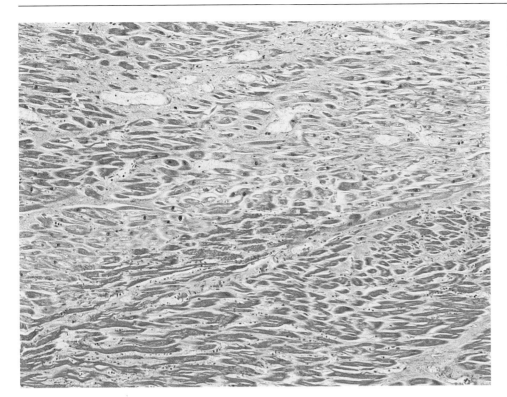

Figure 7.9A. Note the contraction band myonecrosis and interstitial neutrophils.

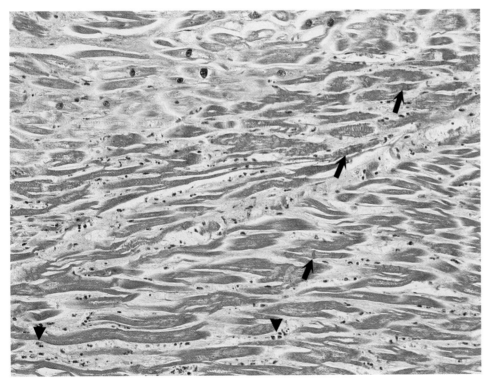

Figure 7.9B. Myocardial infarction (at approximately 12 hours). Segment of myocardium with hypereosinophilic myocytes with contraction band necrosis (arrows) and nascent neutrophilic infiltrate (arrowheads).

Figure 7.10A. Myocardial infarction (at approximately 4–12 hours). Myocardium with early ischemic changes and two geographically distinct populations of myocytes. The myocytes with pink cytoplasm are "normal" and the myocytes which are hypereosinophilic are undergoing ischemic insult and coagulative myocytolysis.

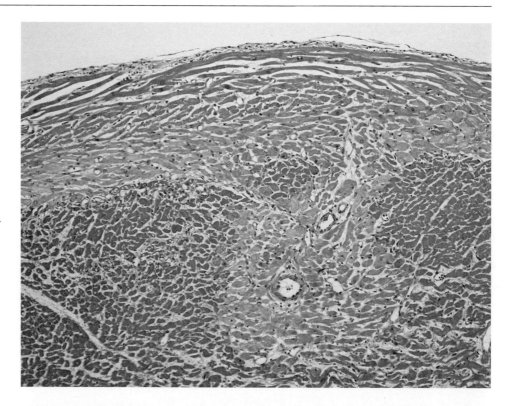

Figure 7.10B. High power reveals contraction-band myonecrosis but no neutrophilic infiltrate as yet.

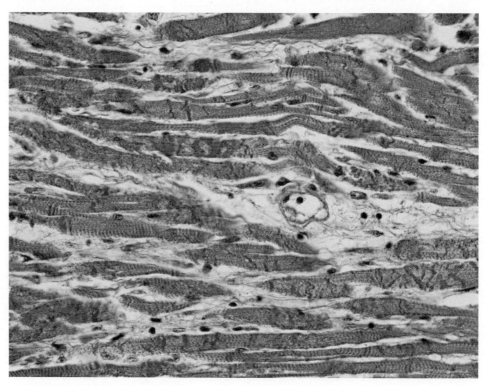

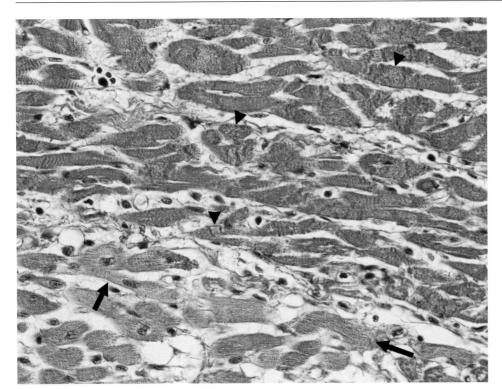

Figure 7.10C. Note border region between relatively "normal" myocytes (arrows) and those undergoing coagulative myocytolysis (arrowheads).

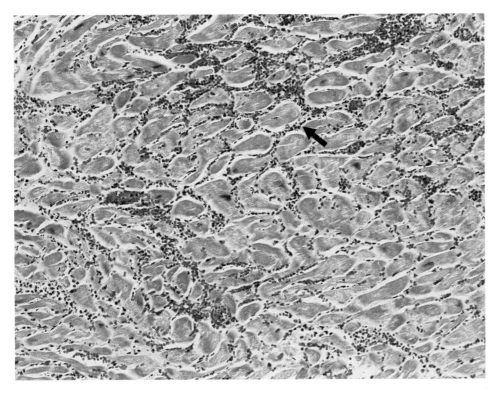

Figure 7.11A. Acute myocardial infarct of the left ventricle. Hemorrhage accompanied by an acute inflammatory infiltrate (arrow). The cardiac myocytes are intensely eosinophilic with focal loss of nuclei, consistent with early coagulative necrosis. The presence of neutrophils and the lack lymphocytes suggest this infarct is approximately 24 hours old.

Figure 7.11B. A higher-power view of the acute myocardial infarct. In this image the neutrophils are quite obvious (arrow).

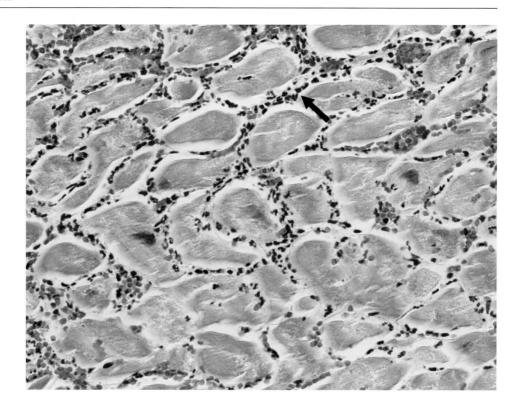

Subacute infarction

Figure 7.12A. Subacute myocardial infarct of the left ventricle with rupture (between arrows) of ventricular wall. There is acute hemorrhage extending from the endocardium to the epicardial adipose tissue. Rupture of the ventricular wall typically occurs 5 to 7 days following a myocardial infarct as a consequence of loss of myocytes from neutrophil and macrophage phagocytosis of necrotic myocyte debris, increased edema and the production of granulation tissue, all of which weaken the ventricular wall in the face of continued high systolic systemic pressures.

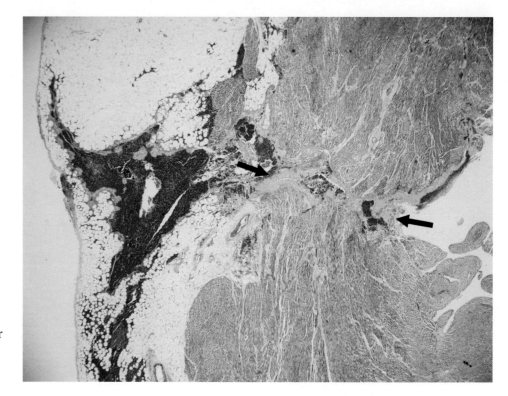

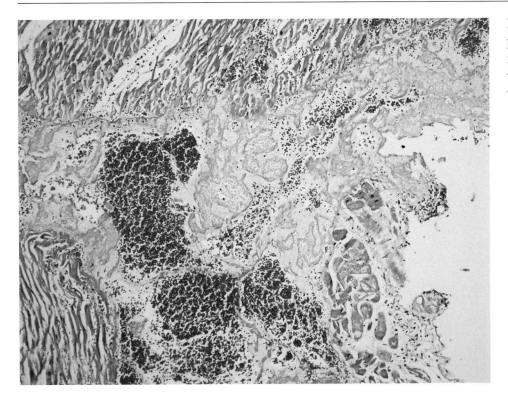

Figure 7.12B. A higher-power view of a subacute myocardial infarct of the left ventricle with rupture of the ventricular wall.

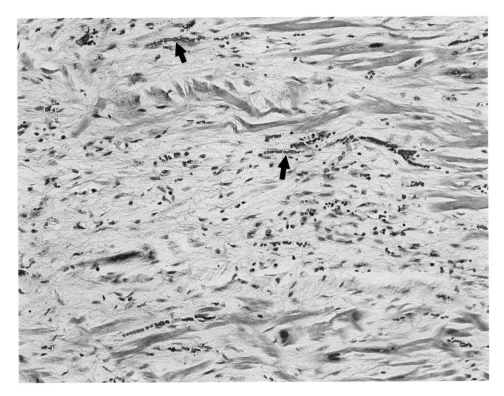

Figure 7.13. Subacute infarct with granulation tissue. There are loosely arranged collagen bundles surrounding several newly formed blood vessels (arrows) at the edge of a myocardial infarct. This histologic appearance becomes prominent around 10 to 14 days.

Figure 7.14A. Subacute myocardial infarction (at approximately 1 week). Myocardium with myocyte degeneration, macrophage infiltration, and nascent loose granulation tissue with neovascularization.

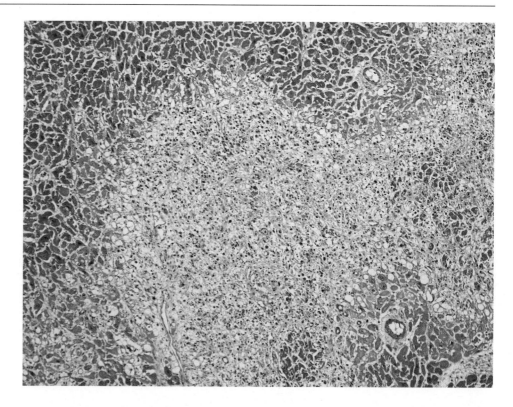

Figure 7.14B. Higher-power revealing angiogenesis (arrowheads) and hemosiderin-laden macrophages (arrows).

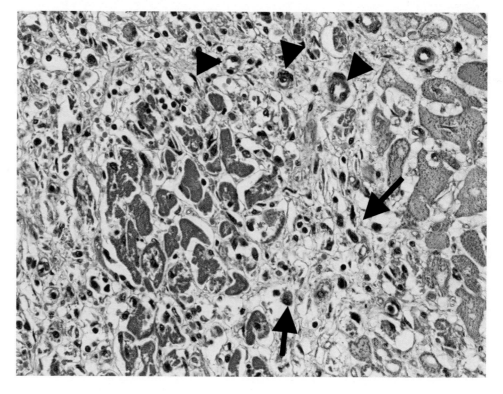

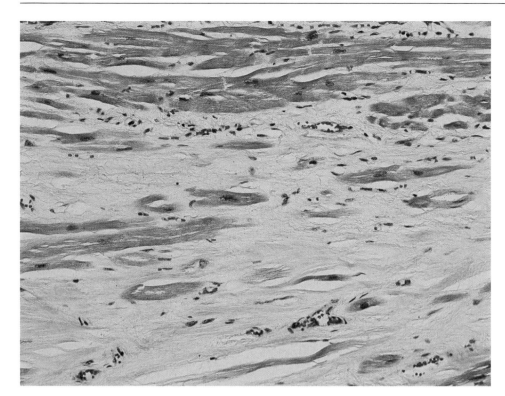

Figure 7.15. Myocardial scar. The end result of the myocardial response to injury is the production of fibrous or "scar" tissue. Once this has occurred it is impossible to age the lesion other than to say it is remote. A number of the surrounding cardiac myocytes contain enlarged nuclei, consistent with hypertension.

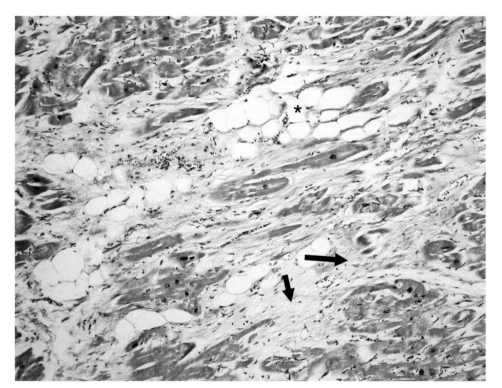

Figure 7.16. Remote myocardial injury. There is increased fibrosis within the interstitium (arrows). One of the late responses of the heart to injury is the conversion of muscle into adipose, sometimes referred to as "fatty metamorphosis" (asterisk). This change is essentially a scar composed of fat and can be arrythymogenic.

Figure 7.17. Remote infarct of the papillary muscle of the left ventricle. There is fibrosis separating viable cardiac myocytes and involving the subendocardial region (arrows). The subendocardium and the papillary muscles are most susceptible to ischemia owing to their tenuous blood supply; therefore, papillary muscles are often scarred.

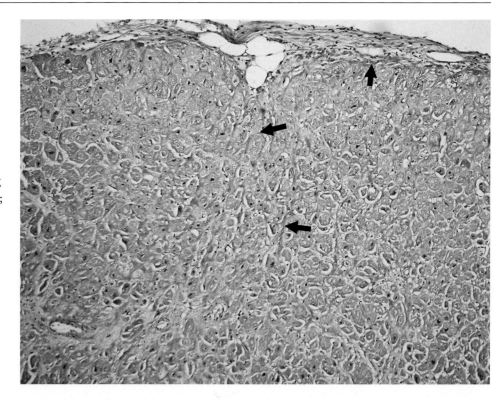

Figure 7.18A. Mummification of cardiac myofibers. Bands of fibrosis separate individual cardiac myocytes. Several of the affected myofibers are shrunken and lack distinct nuclei.

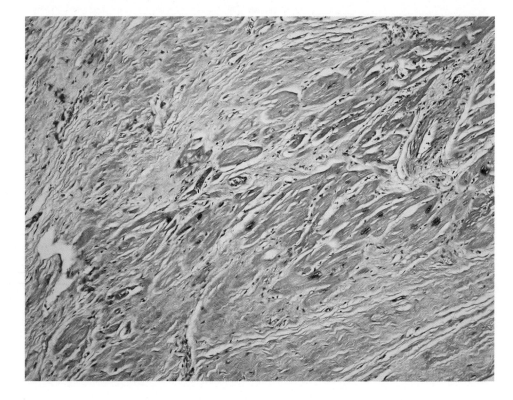

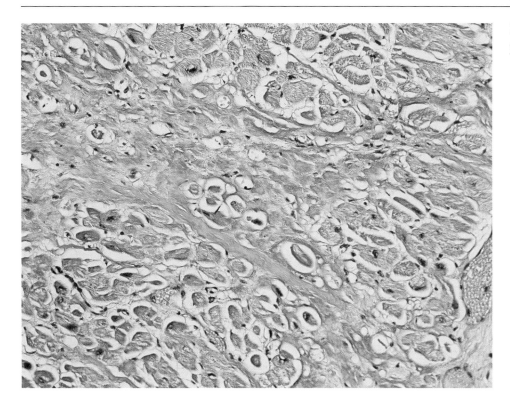

Figure 7.18B. A higher-power view of Figure 7.18A.

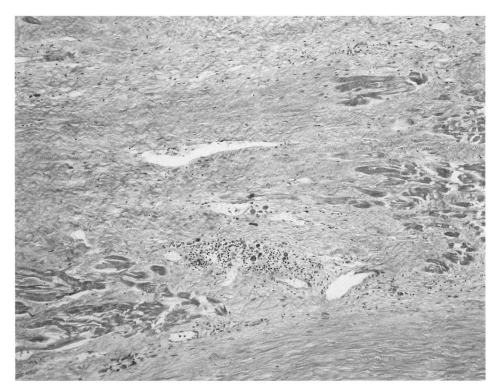

Figure 7.19A. Remote myocardial infarction (at more than 3 weeks). Geographic areas of fibrosis admixed with vascular channels, entrapped myocytes, and hemosiderin-laden macrophages.

Figure 7.19B. Note the
entrapped myocytes
(arrow) and siderophages
(arrowhead)

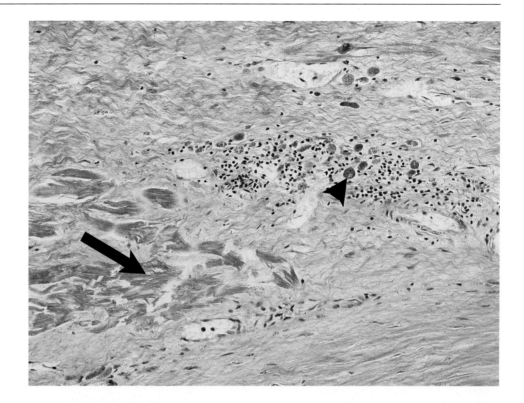

Figure 7.20. Heart after
prolonged cardiopulmonary
resuscitation efforts. There
are multiple foci of acute
hemorrhage (arrow) and
diffuse interstitial edema
(asterisk). This finding can be
differentiated from an acute
myocardial infarct by the lack
of increased eosinophilia,
wavy fibers, contraction
bands and degenerating
cardiac myocytes. Compare
with Figures 7.8A and B.

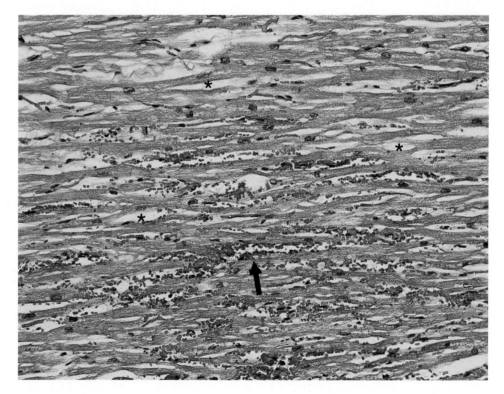

Stigmata of heart failure

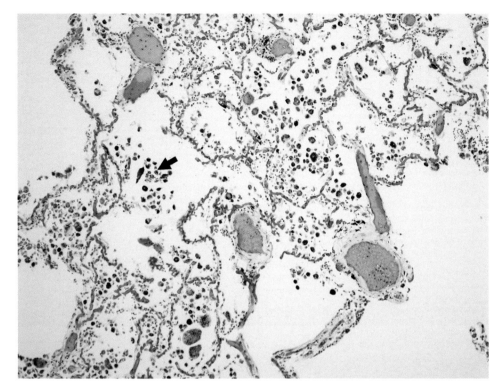

Figure 7.21. Chronic heart failure. There are numerous hemosiderin-laden macrophages present in the alveolar spaces (arrow). This typically appears as a consequence of left-sided heart failure as hemoglobin from erythrocytes is phagocytosed by macrophages and converted into hemosiderin.

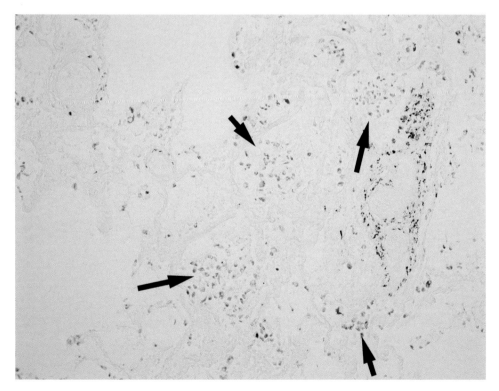

Figure 7.22. Heart failure. Iron stain on lung tissue. Note the blue color (arrows) of the hemosiderin in each of the alveolar macrophages, or so-called "heart failure cells."

Figure 7.23A. Centrilobular necrosis. There is a hemorrhage in the centrilobular region with necrotic perilobular hepatocytes (arrow) surrounded by viable hepatocytes. This morphology is caused by passive chronic congestion.

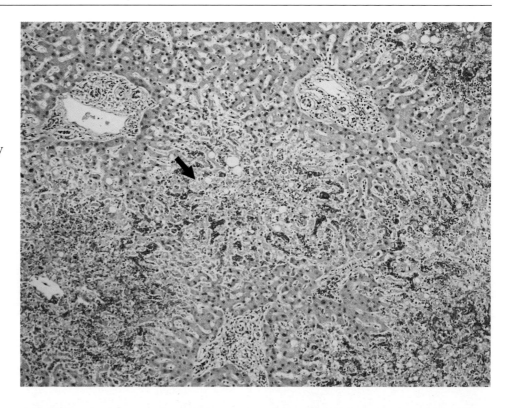

Figure 7.23B. Note the billiary stasis also present (arrows).

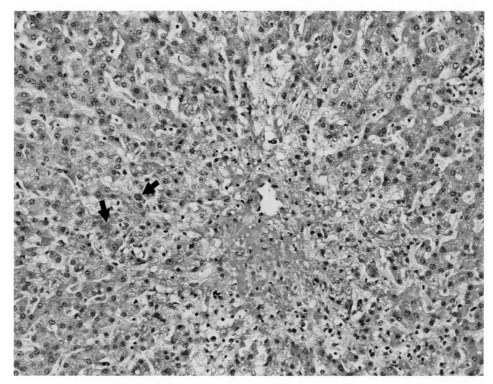

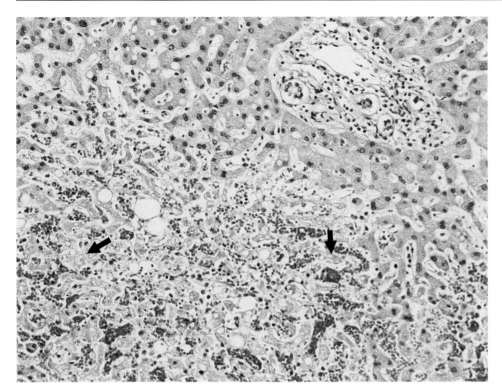

Figure 7.23C. The necrosis (arrows) is easy to see in this high-power view. This commonly occurs because of elevated caval pressures caused by right heart failure and static chronic passive congestion. The gross correlate to this histologic finding is the so-called "nutmeg liver."

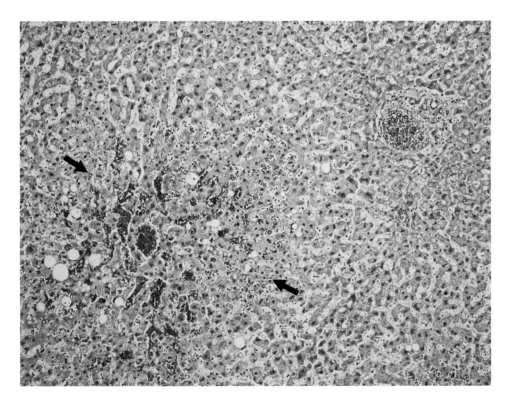

Figure 7.24. Centrilobular congestion. Early in circulatory compromise there is congestion in the perilobular region of the liver (between arrows).

Coronary artery atherosclerosis

Figure 7.25. Atheroma. There is thickening of the intima with proliferation of myofibroblasts (asterisk); cholesterol cleft formation (arrow), and calcium deposition (arrowhead).

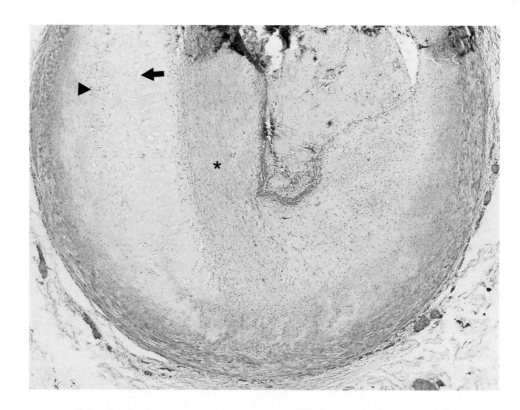

Figure 7.26A. Severe coronary artery atherosclerotic stenosis. Low-power view of a coronary artery with severe luminal stenosis by an atheroma. The media/adventitia commonly manifests chronic inflammation and can demonstrate calcification.

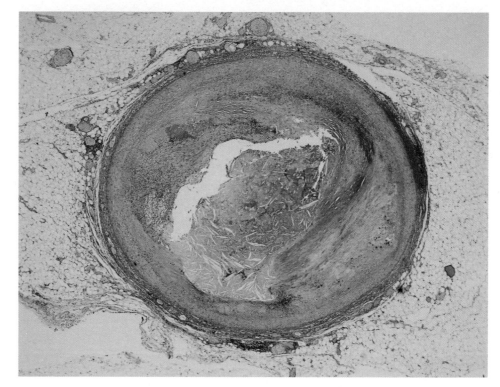

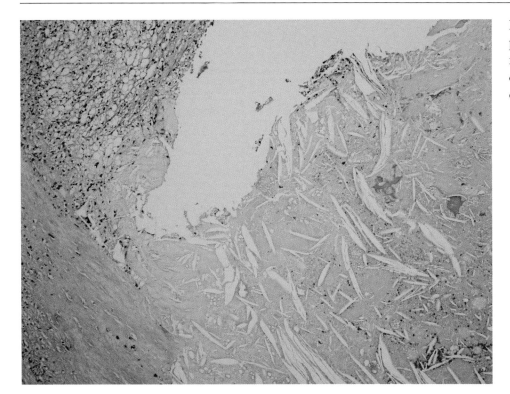

Figure 7.26B. Higher-power view revealing foamy macrophages and plaque with characteristic cholesterol clefts.

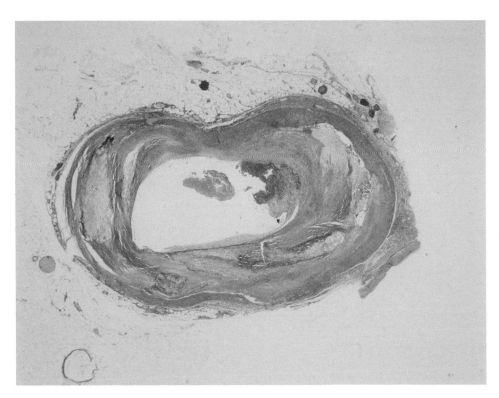

Figure 7.27A. Organizing coronary artery thrombosis. Section of thrombosed coronary artery with adherent blood clot.

Figure 7.27B. Note the fibroblast and endothelial cell in growth (arrow), characteristic of the process of organization. Eventually the erythrocytes will be phagocytized and a collagenous latticework with endothelial-lined canals will result.

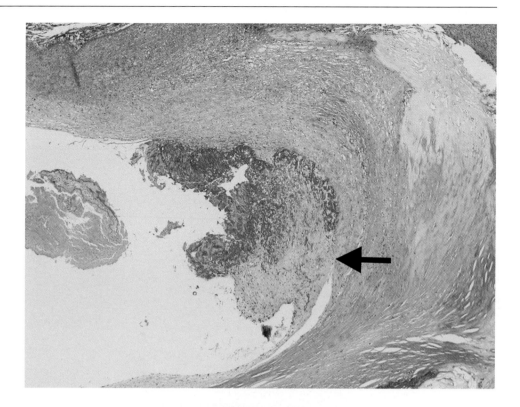

Figure 7.28A. Acute thrombus in coronary artery, following plaque rupture. The intima is thickened and a fibrous cap is present comprised of myofibroblasts and cholesterol clefts (asterisk). Also note the calcium deposits (arrowhead). The plaque has ruptured, inducing the formation of a thrombus. Within the rupture site there is acute hemorrhage and acute inflammation, accompanied by early fibrin deposition (arrow). Dating a thrombus is difficult,; however, a few points bare mentioning. After 12 to 24 hours there is the influx of neutrophils, which peaks at around 3 or 4 days. After 5 to 7 days there is the influx of chronic inflammatory cells. Re- endothelialization, accompanied by the infiltration of fibrous tissue, will appear after a week. The complete organization of the thrombus with recanalization can take up to a month.

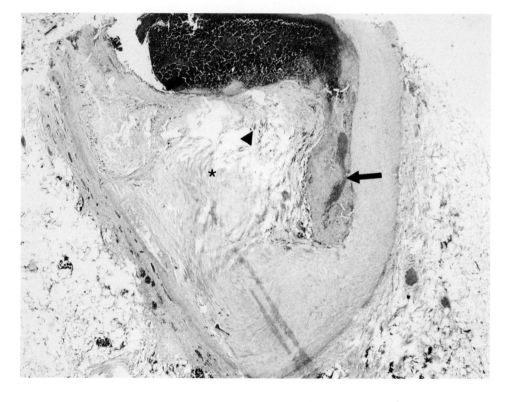

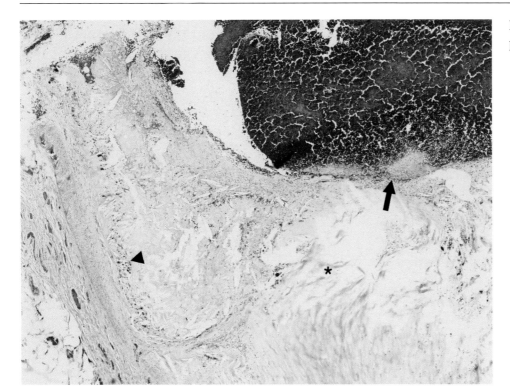

Figure 7.28B. A higher-power view.

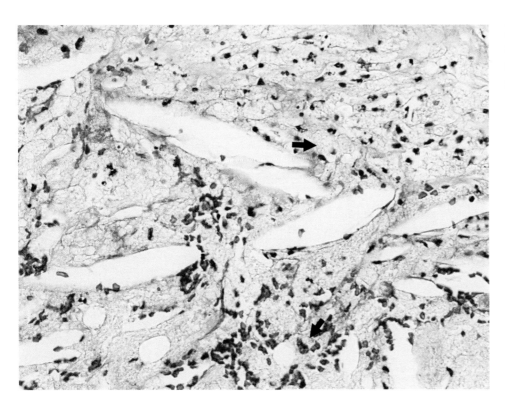

Figure 7.28C. At high magnification one can clearly see the lipid-laden macrophages (arrows).

CEREBRAL VASCULAR SEQUELAE OF HYPERTENSIVE AND ATHEROSCLEROTIC CARDIOVASCULAR DISEASE

Figure 7.29. Hypertensive changes. The artery in this section of white matter is thickened and demonstrates early hyptertensive changes such as perivascular clearing (asterisk) and hemosiderin deposition (arrowhead). There are also corpora amylase present (arrow).

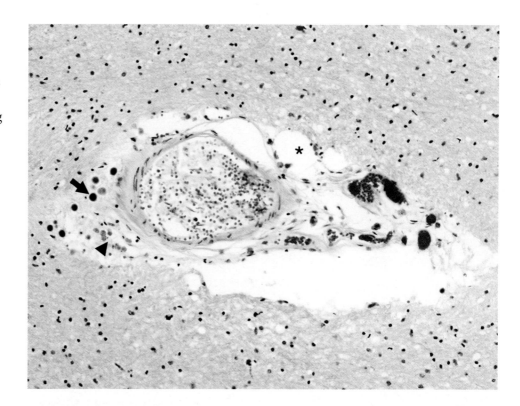

Figure 7.30A. Remote cerebral infarct. There is a remote infarct composed of gliosis and macrophages. Notice the basophilic, black discoloration of the neurons characteristic of mineralization (arrow). Mineralization (also called ferruginization) can be seen as early as one week following an infarct.

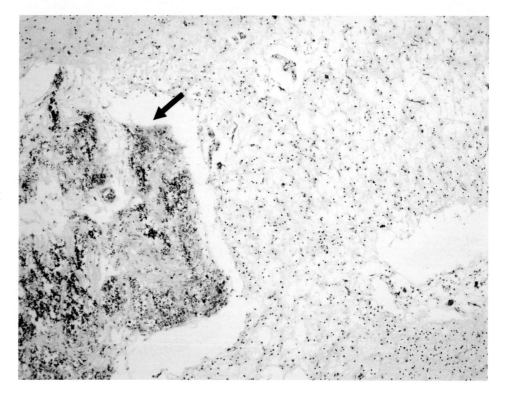

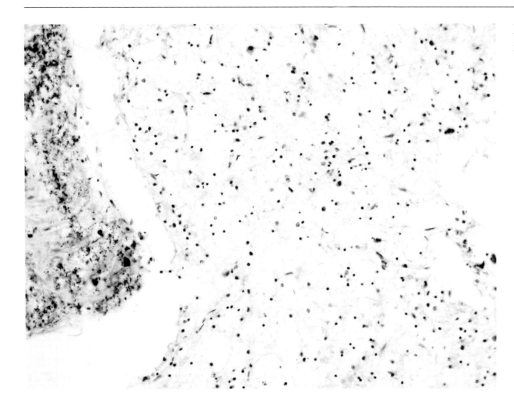

Figure 7.30B. A higher magnification of the infarct.

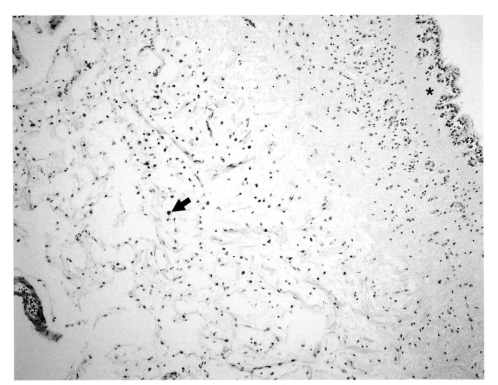

Figure 7.31. Remote lacunar infarct. A glial-lined cyst within the caudate ependymal lining (asterisk) with residual hemosiderin-laden macrophages (arrow). Macrophages may persist for many years. Once a lesion displays this histologic appearance it cannot be dated and is best described as "remote."

Stigmata of cerebral vascular catastrophes

Figure 7.32A. Amyloid angiopathy. This is a haematoxylin and eosin (H&E) section from the occipital lobe. Amyloid angiopathy is unique in that it usually results in a superficial cortical bleed and is most common in the occipital lobe. Note the thick and hyalinized blood vessels in the leptomeninges (arrow). The infarct is remote as evidenced by an intense gliotic reaction and mineralization of neurons (asterisk).

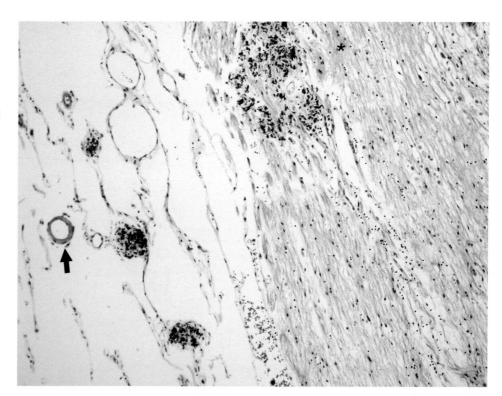

Figure 7.32B. A higher magnification.

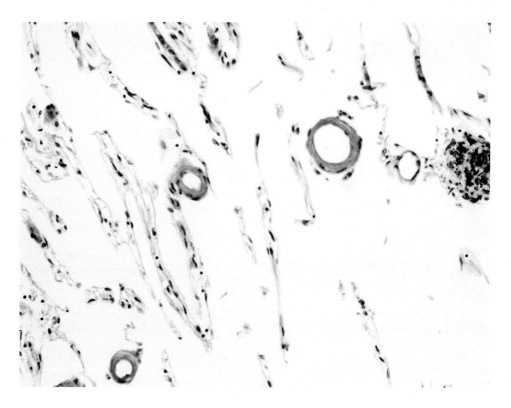

CO

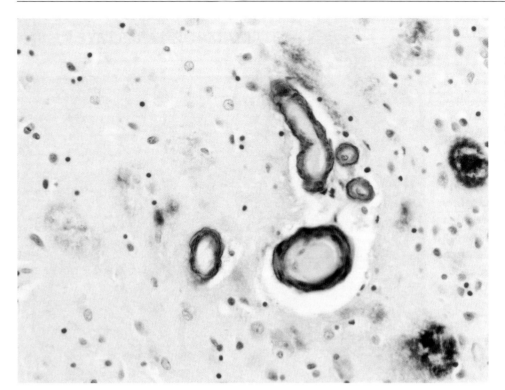

Figure 7.33. Amyloid angiopathy. Beta4 amyloid immunohistochemical staining. This is best appreciated in the leptomeningeal or superficial cortical vasculature. Notice the intense staining within the vessel wall.

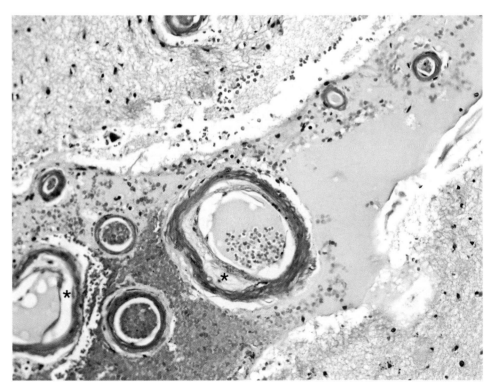

Figure 7.34. Acute cerebral hemorrhage caused by amyloid angiopathy. There is acute hemorrhage within the superficial cortex extending into the subarachnoid space, typical of amyloid angiopathy. The surrounding blood vessels are thickened and hyalinized with a "lumen within a lumen," or "double barrel" appearance (asterisks).

Figure 7.37A. Normal SA node. The SA node (asterisk) abuts the cardiac myocytes of the right atrium and the epicardial adipose tissue superficially (double asterisk). Identification of the sinoatrial nodal artery (arrow) is helpful in locating the SA node.

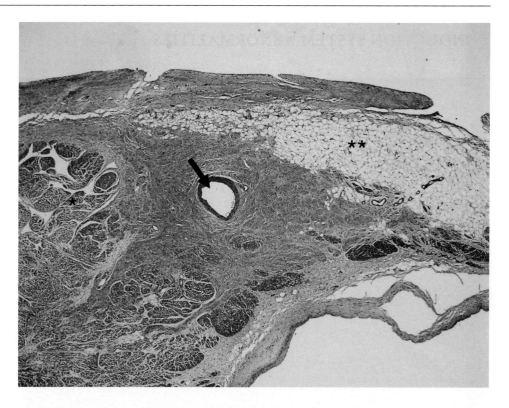

Figure 7.37B. Trichrome stain of normal SA node.

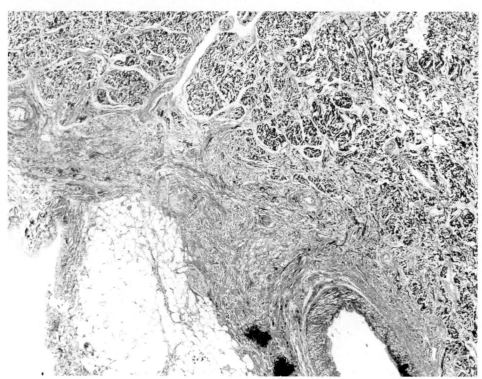

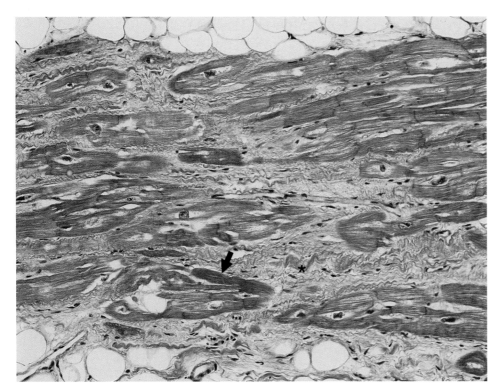

Figure 7.38. Arrhythmogenic right ventricular dysplasia (ARVD). The wall of the right ventricle is thin and is infiltrated by adipose tissue, creating islands of cardiac myocytes (arrow). This condition usually affects young individuals, resulting in sudden death while exercising. The amount of adipose tissue within the ventricles normally increases with age and should not be confused with ARVD. Key to the microscopic diagnosis is the presence of dysplastic residual cardiac myocytes and increased fibrosis (asterisk) within the islands of residual myocardium.

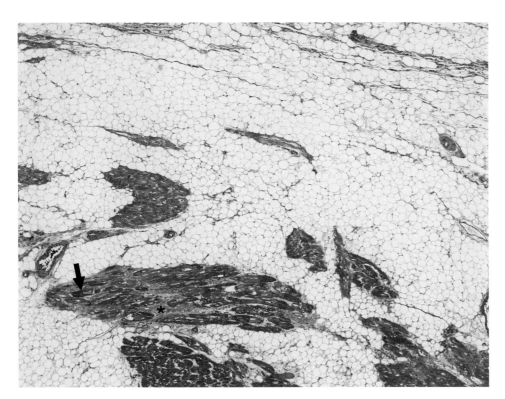

Figure 7.39. ARVD. The wall of the right ventricle is replaced by adipose tissue. The residual islands of myocardial cells demonstrate increased fibrosis (asterisk) and abnormal appearing myocytes (arrow).

HYPERTROPHIC CARDIOMYOPATHY

Figure 7.40. Hypertrophic cardiomyopathy, left ventricle. There is disarray of the overall architecture of the cardiac myocytes. Note the intense fibrosis surrounding the disorganized myofibers that have a "branching" appearance. This 17-year-old individual died suddenly, engaged in a sporting competition. This diagnosis cannot be used simply with an enlarged heart. This is a specific diagnosis with a specific gross impression.

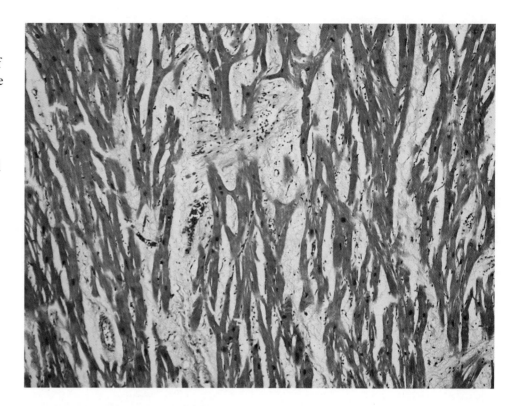

INFILTRATIVE DISEASES

Figure 7.41A. Lymphocytic myocarditis. Often lymphocytic myocarditis is subtle and very focal. In this section there is an increased number of lymphocytes within the interstitium, with early injury to the cardiac myocytes manifested by increased eosinophilia and pyknosis (arrow).

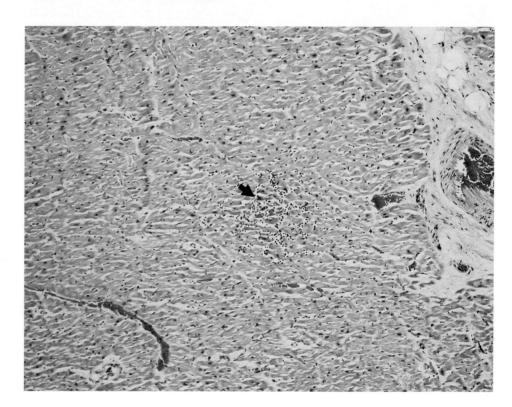

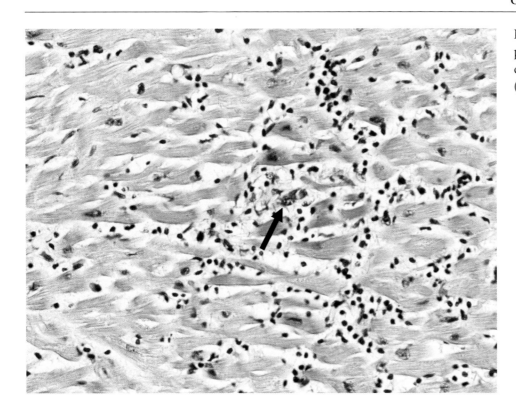

Figure 7.41B. A higher-power view demonstrating a degenerating cardiac myocyte (arrow).

INFLAMMATORY DISEASE

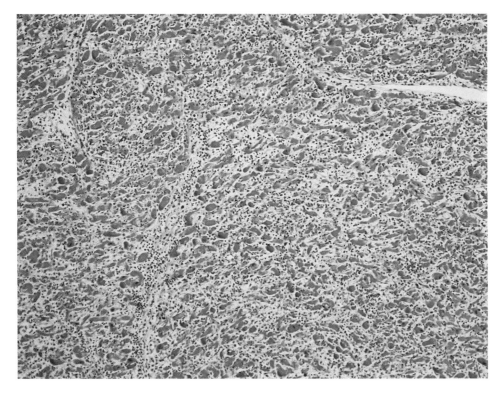

Figure 7.42A. Acute lymphocytic myocarditis. Low-power view of myocardium with florid interstitial chronic inflammatory infiltrate.

Figure 7.42B. Higher-power view highlighting the lymphocytic infiltrate and myocyte degeneration (arrows). Chronic inflammatory activity in the heart can result in interstitial myocardial fibrosis, and the potential for cardiac arrhythmias. Remember, a few lymphocytes in the interstitium does not a myocarditis make. Take extra heart sections, look for lymphocytes and myocyte degeneration. Chronic myocarditis with healing can look very similar to post-ischemic myocardium with markedly elevated interstitial and perivascular fibrosis.

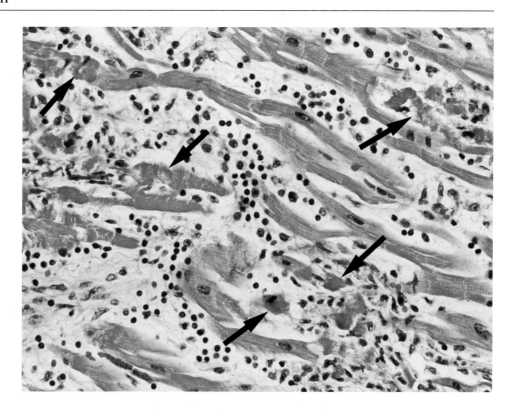

Figure 7.43A. Lymphocytic epicarditis. There are an increased number of lymphocytes (arrow) within the epicardium in conjunction with fibrosis (asterisk). Pericardial inflammation may be the result of cardiac diseases, systemic disorders or as part of a paraneoplastic syndrome.

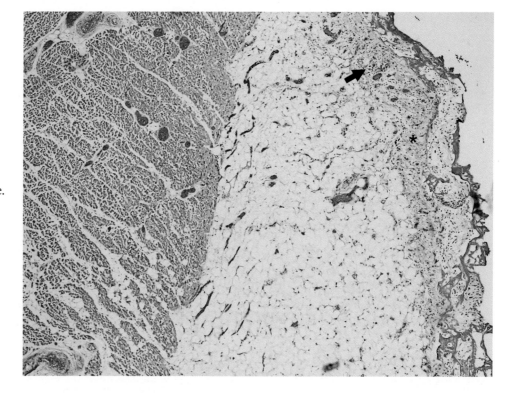

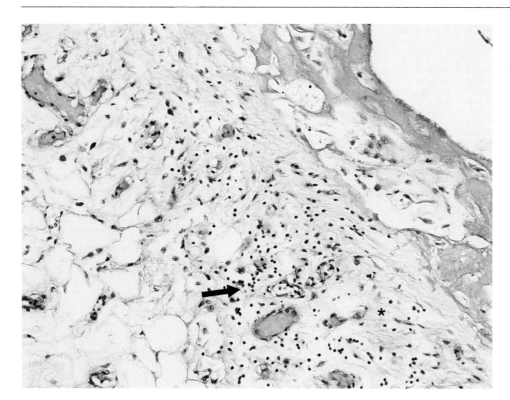

Figure 7.43B. A higher-power view of lymphocytic epicarditis.

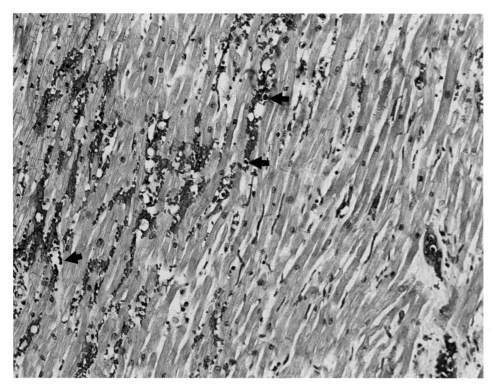

Figure 7.44A. Eosinophilic myocarditis. There are eosinophils infiltrating the myocardium (arrows). Note the acute hemorrhage within the myocardium. The cause of eosinophilic myocarditis is often nebulous. It can be seen in association with hypersensitivity/allergic reactions and infectious processes.

Figure 7.44B. A higher-power view.

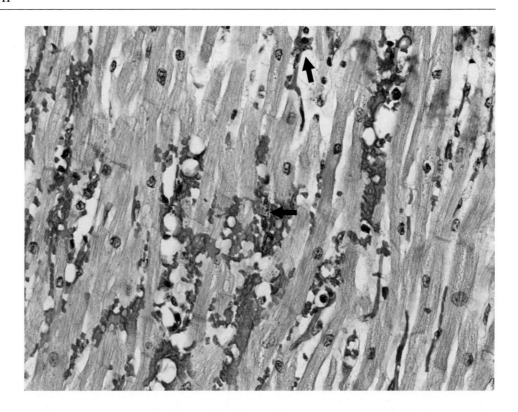

Figure 7.44C. Edema and eosinophils (arrows) infiltrating the myocardium.

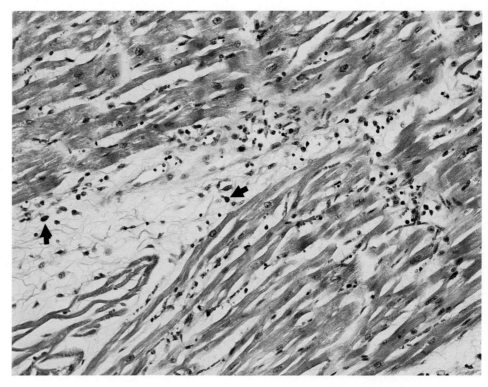

EPILEPSY

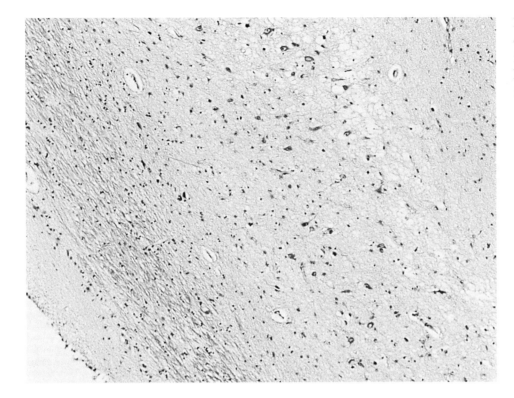

Figure 7.45. Hippocampus in epilepsy. The loss of neurons in the CA-1 region of the hippocampus. Notice the increased space between cells.

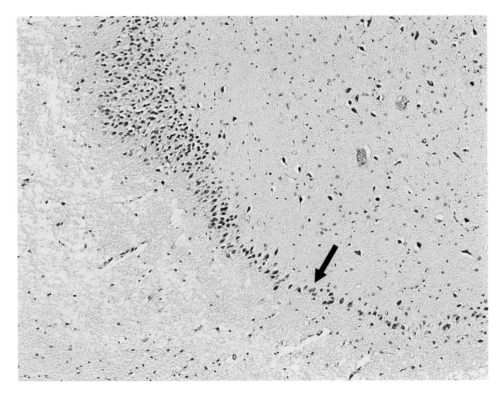

Figure 7.46. Dentate gyrus in epilepsy. There is neuronal loss manifested by thinning of the dentate gyrus (arrow).

Figure 7.47. Hippocampus stained with glial fibrillary acidic protein (GFAP). Notice the increased staining in the CA-4 region of Ammon's horn. The astrocytic processes are also creeping between the neurons of the dentate gyrus. Increased GFAP staining within the CA-1 and CA-4 regions of the hippocampus, along with increased subpial staining are common but non-specific findings in epilepsy.

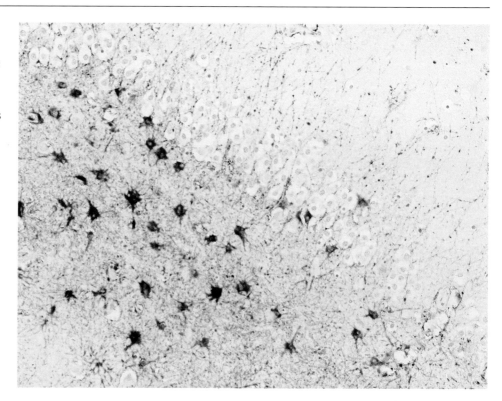

Figure 7.48A. Pinocytoma. A pinocytoma that lead to epilepsy in a 28-year-old male who died as a result of the seizure. The tumor is surrounded by a layer of reactive astrocytes (arrow) and there is calcification within the mass (asterisk). This is a rare cause of epilepsy.

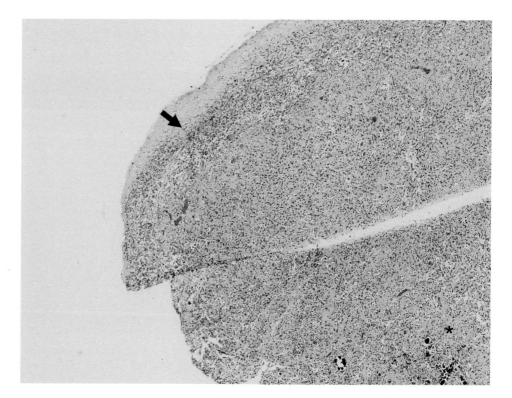

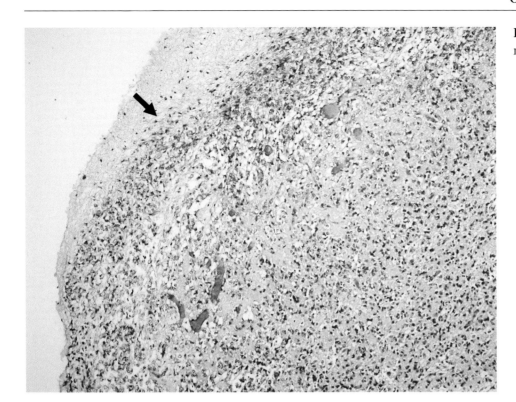

Figure 7.48B. A higher magnification of the lesion.

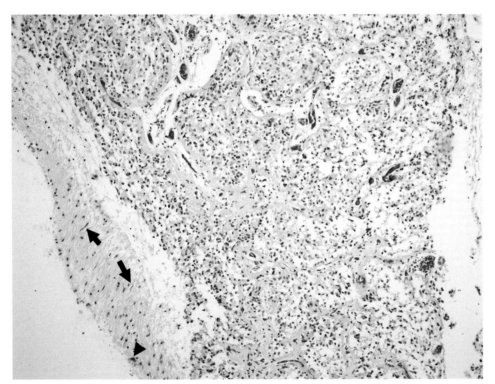

Figure 7.49A. Pinocytoma. This lesion can be differentiated from normal pineal gland by the piloid astroglial process and Rosenthal fibers surrounding the mass (arrows). Often granular bodies are seen (arrowhead). Pineocytomas are usually solid rather than cystic and maintain an organoid appearance.

Figure 7.49B. A higher magnification of these features.

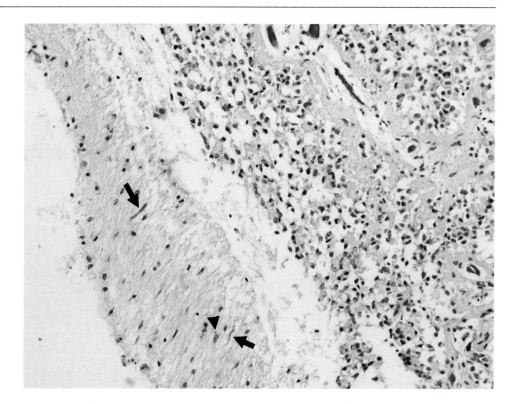

Figure 7.50. Capillary telangiectasia. There is a collection of dilated capillaries that are separated from one another by brain parenchyma. Often these lesions are located in the brainstem or pons but can be found in the cerebral hemispheres, cerebellum, and spinal cord. They are typically an incidental finding, but can be associated with seizures or hemorrhage.

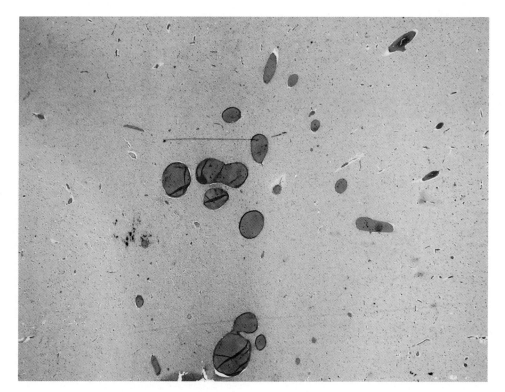

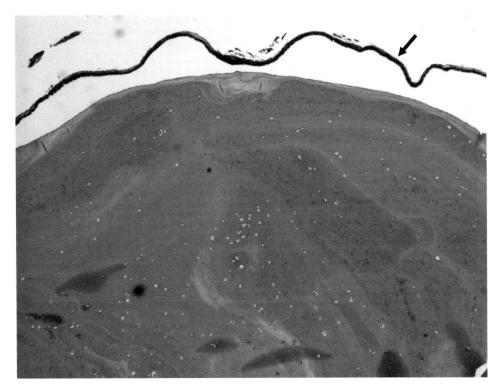

Figure 7.51A. Colloid cyst of the third ventricle. There is a thin cyst wall (arrow) covering the pink colloid contents (asterisk). Though not associated with epilepsy, colloid cysts can be a cause of sudden death if there is an acute blockage of the interventricular foramina resulting in acute hydrocephalus (photograph courtesy of Dr. Brian Moore, Springfield, IL).

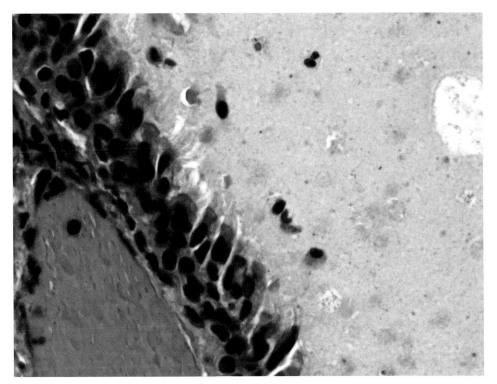

Figure 7.51B. A higher magnification of the colloid cyst demonstrates the cuboidal epithelium of the cyst wall. Occasionally, secretory vacuoles can be seen just under the epithelium (not seen in this photograph) (photograph courtesy of Dr. Brian Moore, Springfield, IL).

DIABETES MELLITUS

Figure 7.52. Nodular diabetic glomerulosclerosis. There is nodular sclerosis of the glomeruli, known as Kimmelstiel – Wilson lesions.

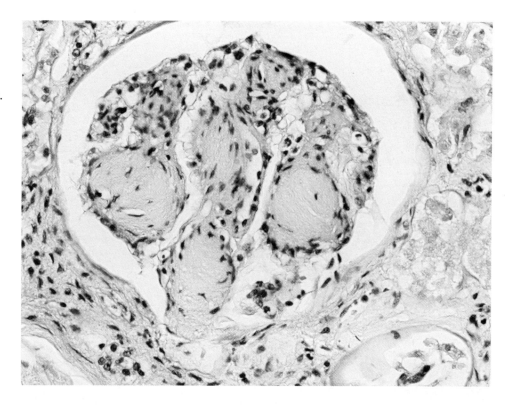

ALLERGY

Figure 7.53A. Anaphylaxis. This section of larynx demonstrates intense edema, creating clear spaces between the strands of connective tissue (asterisk) with focal inflammation (arrow).

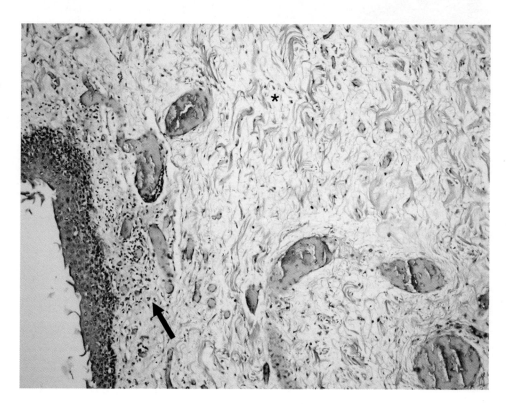

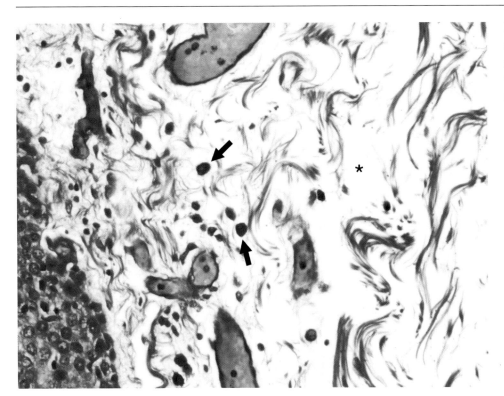

Figure 7.53B. A higher-spower view demonstrates numerous mast cells (arrow) within the edematous tissue (asterisk).

PULMONARY

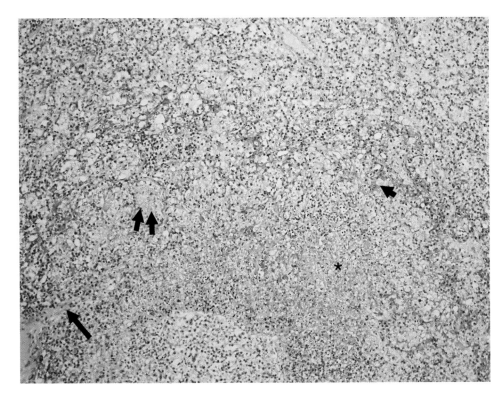

Figure 7.54A. Organizing diffuse alveolar damage. There are alveoli filled with proteinaceous material (double arrow), hyaline membranes (short arrow) and macrophages. Also prominent in this section are foci of chronic inflammation, necrosis (asterisk), and early fibrosis (long arrow).

Figure 7.54B. This higher-power view shows a focus of fibroblastic proliferation.

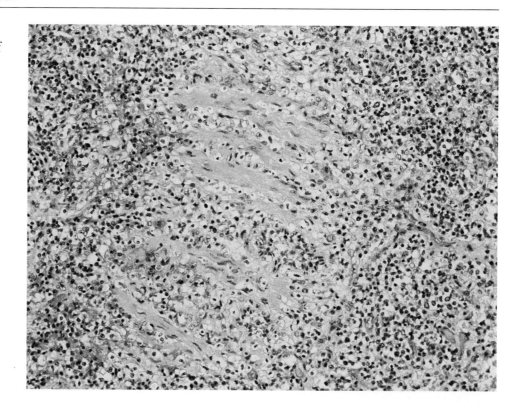

Figure 7.54C. A higher-power view demonstrates many macrophages (arrow).

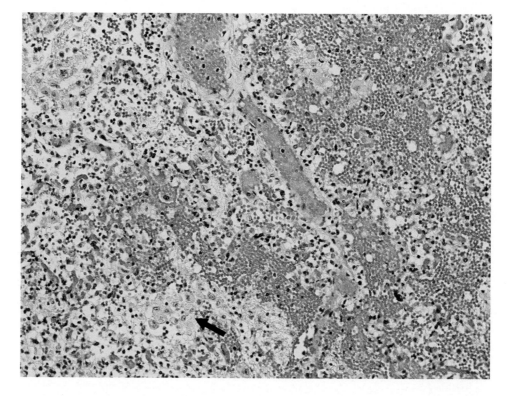

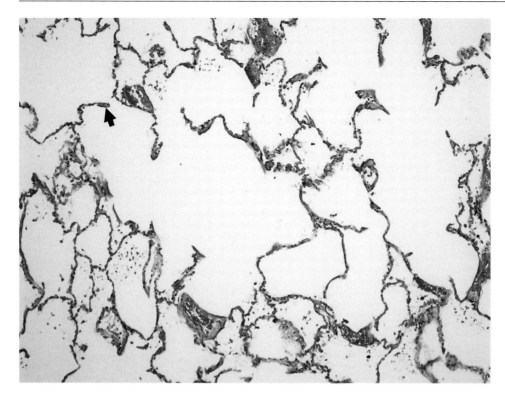

Figure 7.55. Pulmonary hypertension. There is thickening of the arteriole wall, similar to that seen in atherosclerotic cardiovascular disease. Emphysematous changes are also seen in this section; notice the "tennis racquet" or "clubbed"-appearing ends of the disrupted alveolar wall (arrow). Foci of fibrosis are noted throughout the lung. These findings suggest chronic obstructive pulmonary disease as the cause of the pulmonary hypertension.

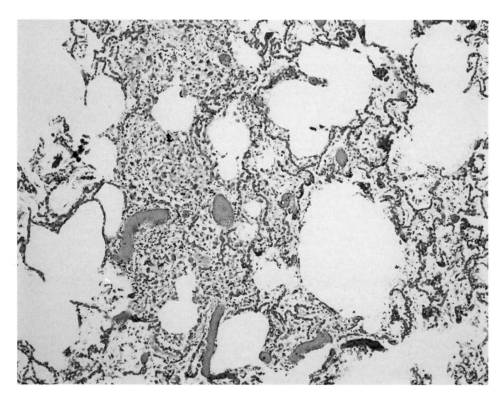

Figure 7.56. Smoker's lung. Common findings in smokers include increased chronic inflammation, desquamated pneumocytes, and carbon deposition, which resemble respiratory bronchiolitis.

Figure 7.57. Fatal pulmonary hemorrhage. The alveolar spaces are completely filled with hemorrhage. Notice the early fibroblastic response (long arrow) and the multiple foci of macrophages (short arrow).

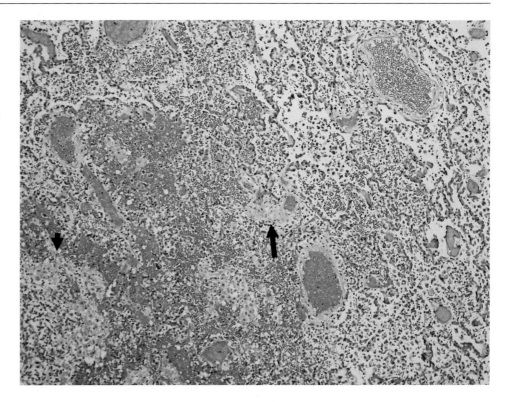

ASTHMA

Figure 7.58. Asthma. There is an exuberant acute and chronic inflammatory infiltrate with a predominance of eosinophils. Also note the thickened basement membrane and the hypertrophied smooth muscle. (Photograph courtesy of Steven Cina, Ft. Lauderdale, FL.)

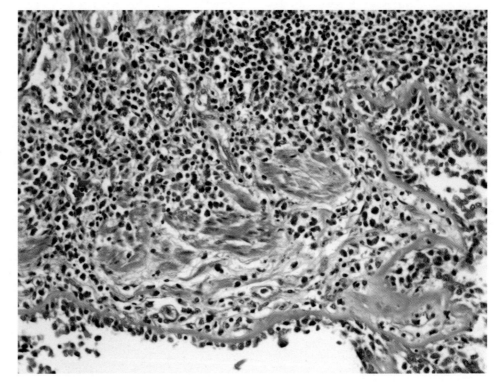

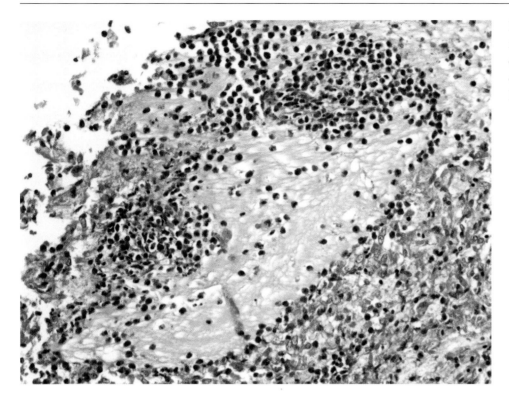

Figure 7.59. There is a mucus plug with abundant eosinophils. (Photograph courtesy of Steven Cina, Ft. Lauderdale, FL.)

SICKLE CELL DISEASE

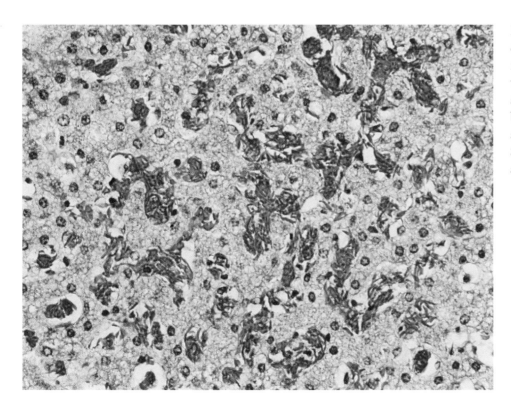

Figure 7.60. Sickle cell disease in the liver. Close inspection of the blood within the congested sinusoids demonstrates red blood cells that are spindle-shaped with pointed ends. Some of the red blood cells are sickled.

Figure 7.61. Sickle cell disease in the lung. The red blood cells in the small arterioles demonstrate balls of red blood cells that are spindle-shaped with pointed ends. Some of the red blood cells are sickled.

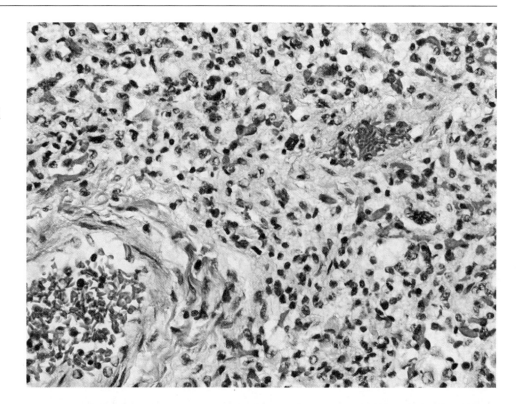

Figure 7.62. Sickle cell disease in the spleen. Later in life the spleen of an individual who has suffered multiple sickle cell attacks will be shrunken and fibrotic. In children, the spleen may show expansion of the red pulp, seen here as the diffuse red coloring of the spleen.

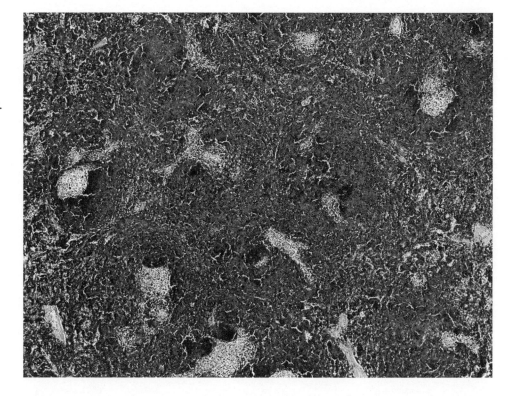

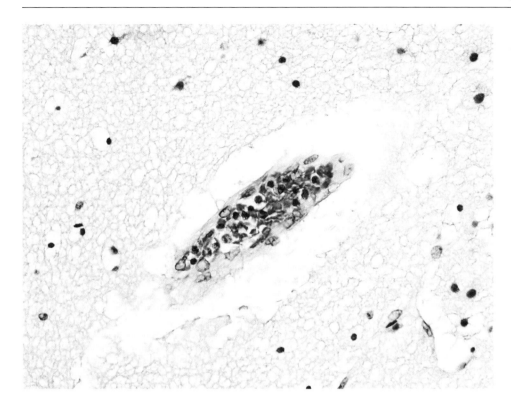

Figure 7.63. Sickle cell disease in the brain. There is cerebral edema surrounding a small artery packed with sickled red blood cells.

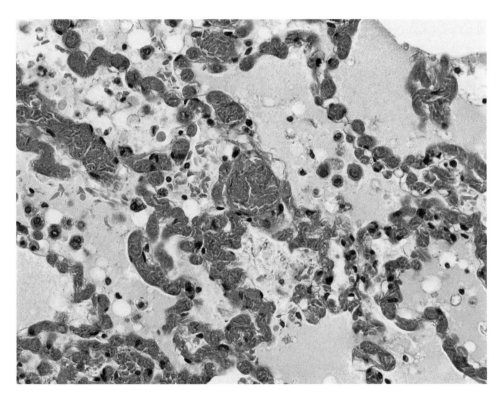

Figure 7.64A. Sickle cell disease. Pulmonary vasculature filled with sickled erythrocytes.

Figure 7.64B. Renal vasculature filled with sickled erythrocytes.

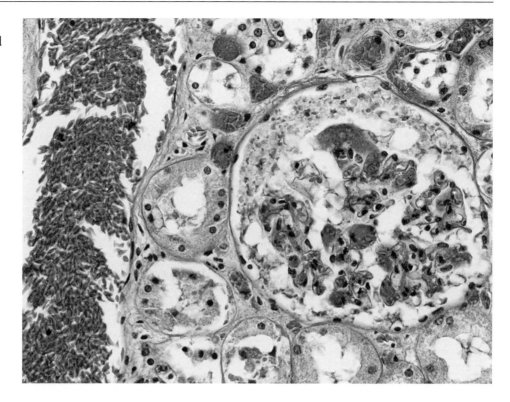

MISCELLANEOUS INFECTIOUS/INFLAMMATORY DISEASE

Figure 7.65. Acute bronchopneumonia. There is an acute inflammatory infiltrate filling the alveolar spaces.

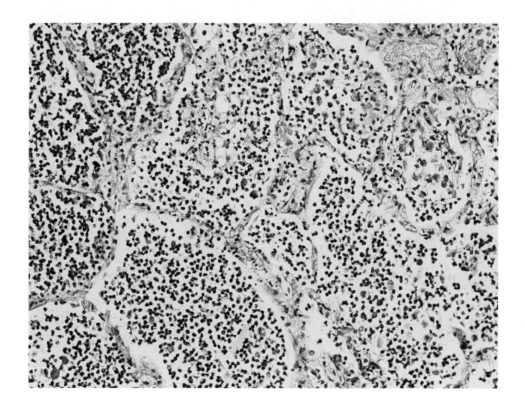

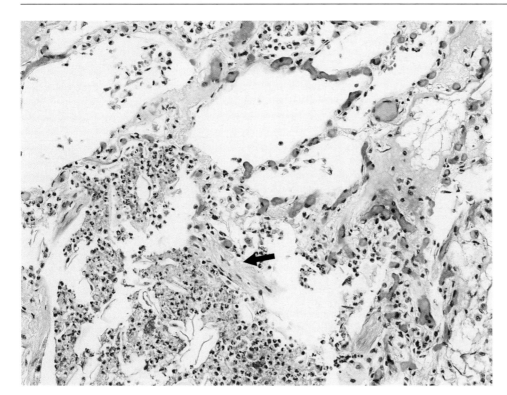

Figure 7.66A. Organizing bronchopneumonia. There is residual acute inflammation, that is beginning to break down, surrounded by regions of fibroblastic proliferation (arrow).

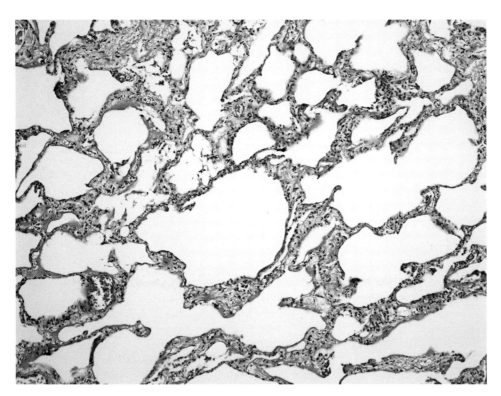

Figure 7.66B. At lower magnification one can see that the alveolar septae are thickened and hypercellular, reflecting early fibrosis.

Figure 7.66C. A higher-power view shows the increased number of fibroblasts within the alveolar septae (arrow).

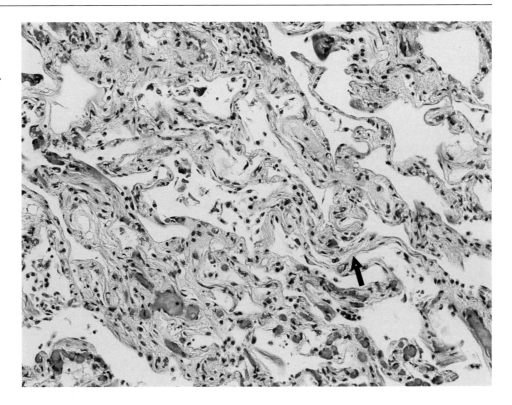

Figure 7.67. Acute bacterial meningitis. There is an extensive acute inflammatory infiltrate present within the leptomeninges.

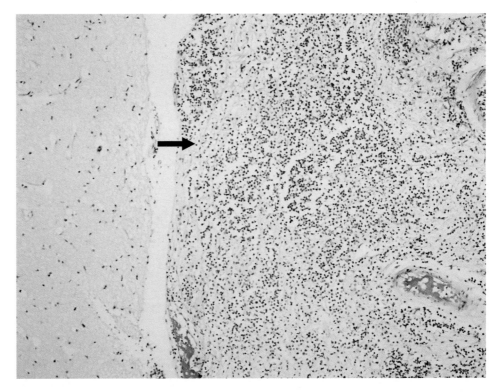

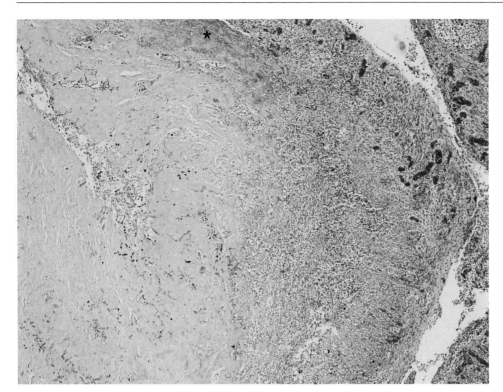

Figure 7.68A. Inflammation of the urinary bladder. There are regions of acute hemorrhage with a neutrophilic infiltrate. Abundant bacterial elements are also visible as a purple "smudge" (asterisk). Also present are multiple foci of chronic inflammation with granulation tissue and giant cell formation.

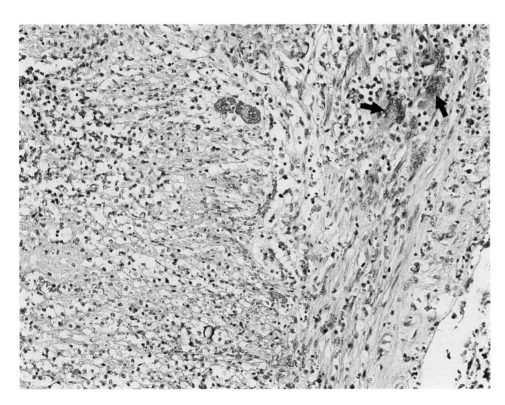

Figure 7.68B. Careful inspection reveals numerous hyphe and spores (arrows).

Figure 7.68C. At higher magnification one can easily see the changes consistent with a fungal infection (arrows).

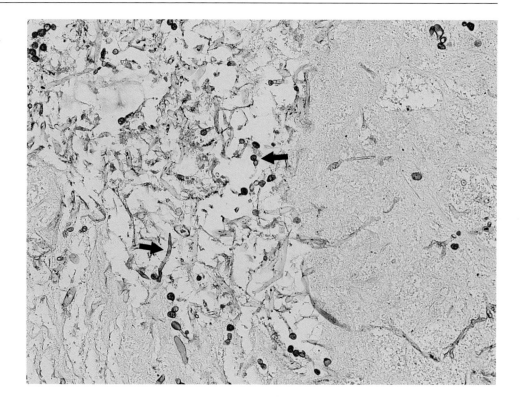

Figure 7.69. Diffuse white-matter loss following cytomegalovirus (CMV) infection. There is rarefaction and vacuolization (asterisk) of the white matter of the basis pontis. No viral inclusions are seen.

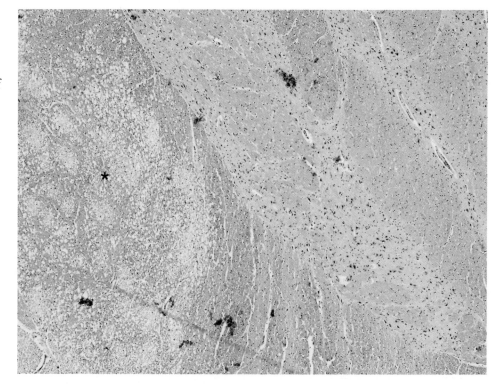

ACQUIRED IMMUNE DEFICIENCY SYNDROME

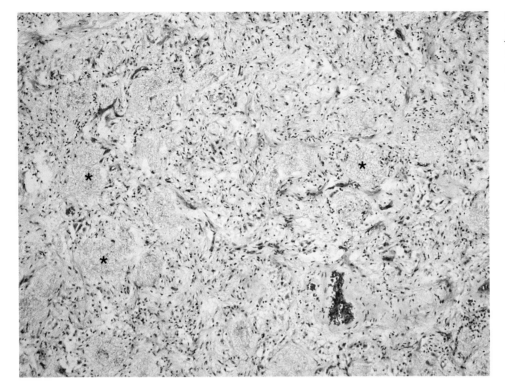

Figure 7.70. *Pneumocystis jirovecii* pneumonia. The alveolar spaces are filled with a foamy proteinaceous exudate (asterisks).

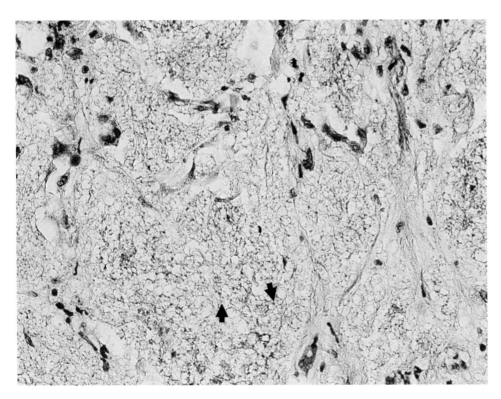

Figure 7.71. Careful inspection will detect small, round *Pneumocystis jirovecii* organisms (arrows).

Figure 7.72. Higher-power photograph of the silver stain from Figure 7.71. The silver stain highlights extensive involvement of the lung by *Pneumocystis jirovecii* pneumonia. The alveolar spaces are filled with organisms.

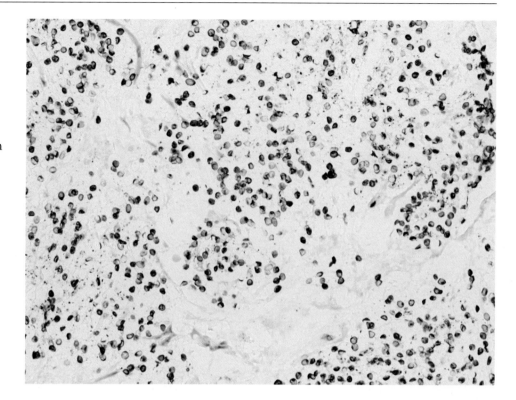

Figure 7.73. Kaposi sarcoma. A proliferation of irregularly shaped blood vessels.

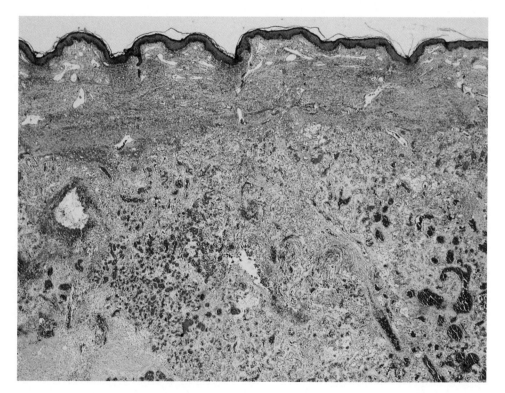

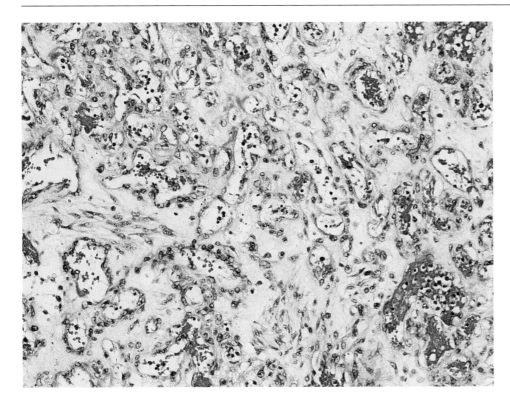

Figure 7.74. Kaposi sarcoma. There is extensive proliferation of perivascular spindle cells.

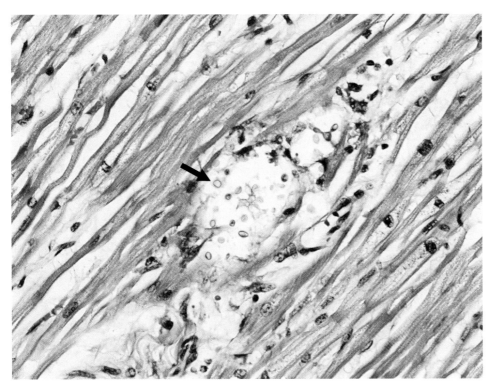

Figure 7.75. Cryptococcus infection of the heart. There are numerous cryptococcus organisms infiltrating the myocardium in this section of left ventricle (arrow).

SUGGESTED READING

Cardiac

Demellawy, E.L., Nasr, A., Alowami, S. An updated review on the clinicopathologic aspects of arrhythmogenic right ventricular cardiomyopathy. *Am J Forensic Med Pathol.* 2009; **30**(1): 78–83.

Gulino, S.P. Examination of the cardiac conduction system: forensic application in cases of sudden death. *Am J Forensic Med Pathol.* 2003; **24**(3): 227–238.

Ottaviani, O., Lavezzi, A.M., Matturri, L. Sudden unexpected death in young athletes. *Am J Forensic Med Pathol.* 2008; **29**(4): 337–349.

Song, Y., Zhu, J., Laaksonen, H., Saukko, P. A. modified method for examining the cardiac conduction system. *Forensic Sci International.* 1997; **86**: 135–138.

Turan, A.A., Karayel, F., Elif, U., *et al.* Sudden death due to eosinophilic endomyocardial diseases: three case reports. *Am J Forensic Med Pathol.* 2008; **29**(4): 354–357.

Veinot, J.P., Johnson, B., Acharya, V., Healey, J. Spectrum of intramyocardial small vessel disease associated with sudden death. *J Forensic Sci.* 2002; **47**(2): 384–388.

Epilepsy

Dube, C.M., Brewster, A.L., Baram, T.Z. Febrile seizures: mechanisms and relationship to epilepsy. *Brain and Development.* 2009; **31**: 366–371.

Englander, J., Bushnik, T., Wright, J.M., Amison, L., Duong, T.T. Mortality in late post-traumatic seizures. *J Neurotrauma.* 2009; **26**: 1471–1477.

Fornes, P., Ratel, S., Lecomte, D. Pathology of arrhythmogenic right ventricular cardio-myopathy/dysplasia: an autopsy study of 20 forensic cases. *J Forensic Sci.* 1998; **43**(4): 777–783.

Mandera, M., Marcol, W., Bierzyńka-Macyszyn, G., Kluczewska, E. Pineal cysts in childhood. *Childs Nerv Syst.* 2003; **19**(10–11) 750–755.

Manno, E.M., Pfeifer, E.A., Cascino, G.D., *et al.* Cardiac pathology in status epilepticus. *Ann Neurol.* 2005; **58**: 954–957.

Reid, A.Y., Galic, M.A., Teskey, G.C., Pittman, Q.J. Febrile seizures: current views and investigations. *Can J Neurol Sci.* 2009; **36**: 679–686.

Shields, L.B., Hunsaker, D.M., Hunsacker, J.C. 3rd, Parker, J.C. Jr. Sudden unexpected death in epilepsy. *Am J Forensic Med Pathol.* 2002; **23**(4): 307–314.

Thom, M. The autopsy in sudden unexpected adult death: epilepsy. *Current Diag Pathol.* 2007; **13**: 389–400.

Pediatrics

Rickert, C.h., Grob, O., Nolte, K.W., *et al.* Leptomeningeal neurons are common findings in infants and are increased in sudden infant death syndrome. *Acta Neuropathol.* 2009; **117**: 275–282.

Thogmartin, J.R., Wilson, C.I., Palma, N.A., Ignacio, S.S., Pellan, W.A. Histologic diagnosis of sickle cell trait: a blinded analysis. *Am J Forensic Med Pathol.* 2009; **30**(1): 36–39.

INTRODUCTION

There are few areas in forensic pathology that are as challenging as deaths involving children. It takes many years of experience to become comfortable with the histology associated with pediatric cases. The normal infant lung is more cellular than the adult and often it is atelectatic, giving the appearance of an inflammatory process. The kidney also is more cellular, and often sclerotic glomeruli are seen as part of the normal development process. These findings can sometimes be confusing. The issues surrounding potential child abuse cases are some of the most difficult we encounter. Trying to determine if an injury is inflicted or accidental is often a challenge and the literature is fraught with inconsistencies. There are also instances where the time of death becomes an issue, such as in fetal demise. This chapter touches on a few of these points and will serve as a guide for this murky, confusing area of forensic pathology. We draw our conclusions from recent publications and hope that the suggested reading section will aid the reader in making up his or her own mind. The autopsy in these cases is just a single piece of information. It must be interpreted in context with a thorough scene investigation, review of complete medical records, and review of all relevant investigative reports such as those written by police or child welfare investigators.

FETAL DEMISE (HOW LONG *IN UTERO* AFTER DEATH)

Table 8.1 Estimating time of death in stillborn fetuses.

Histologic evaluation of fetal organs [1].	
Death-to-delivery time	*Microscopic features*
>4 hours	**Kidney**: Loss (any cell) of cortical tubular nuclear basophilia (G)
>24 Hours	**Liver**: Loss (any cell) of hepatocyte nuclear basophilia (G) **Myocardium**: Inner half (any cell in the endocardium) loss of nuclear basophilia (G) **Adrenal gland**: Cortical (any cell) loss of nuclear basophilia (I)
>36 Hours	**Pancreas**: Maximal (cells of entire organ) loss of nuclear basophilia (I)
>48 Hours	**Myocardium**: Outer half (any cell in the epicardium) loss of nuclear basophilia (G)
>96 Hours	**Bronchus**: Loss (any cell) of epithelial nuclear basophilia (G) **Liver**: Maximal (cells of entire organ) loss of nuclear basophilia (G)
>1 week	**GI tract**: Maximal (cells of entire tract) loss of nuclear basophilia (G) **Adrenal gland**: Maximal (entire organ) loss of nuclear basophilia (G) **Trachea**: Chondrocyte (any cell) loss of nuclear basophilia (G)
>2 weeks	**Lung**: Alveolar wall (any interstitial or alveolar epithelial cell) loss of nuclear basophilia (I)
>4 weeks	**Kidney**: Maximal (cells of entire organ) loss of nuclear basophilia (G)

Nuclear basophilia was superior to the other features assessed because:
- it can be more objectively measured [1], and/or
- it is more strongly associated with time of fetal death than other features [1]

(G): Good predictor; (I): Intermediate predictor

Histologic evaluation of the placenta [2], [3].

Death-to-delivery time	Microscopic features (G)
>6 Hours	Intravascular (leukocyte and endothelial cell) karyorrhexis (>5%)
>48 Hours	Multifocal (10–25%) stem vessel luminal abnormalities (i.e., fibroblast septation of lumina and fibrous luminal obliteration)
>2 weeks	Extensive (>25%) stem vessel luminal abnormalities. Extensive (>25%) villous fibrosis

(G): Good predictor. No histologic placental alterations correlating with time of death (i.e., intravascular karyorrhexis, stem vessel luminal abnormalities, or villous fibrosis) were found to be influenced by length of refrigeration time before fixation [2]. However, after 1–2 weeks of refrigeration, endothelial cells were found floating, both individually and in sheets within vascular lumina [2].

Source:

[1] Genest, D.R., Williams, M.A., Green, M.F. Estimating the time of death in stillborn fetuses, I: histologic evaluation of fetal organs – an autopsy study of 150 stillborns. *Obstet Gynecol* (1992) **80**, 575–584.

[2] Genest, D.R. Estimating the time of death in stillborn fetuses, II: histologic evaluation of the placenta – a study of 71 stillborns. *Obstet Gynecol* (1992), **80**, 585–592.

[3] Marchetti, D., Belviso, M., Marino, M., Gaudio, R. Evaluation of the placenta in a stillborn fetus to estimate the time of death. *Am J Forensic Med Path* (2007), **28**, 38–43.

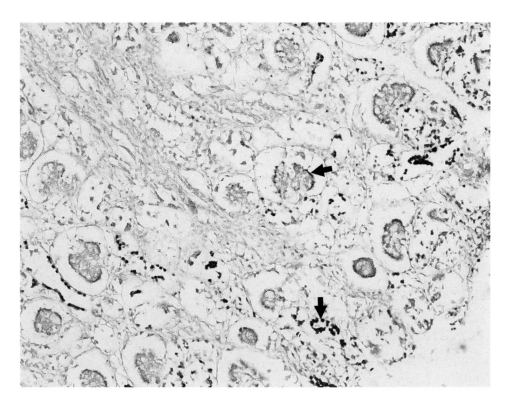

Figure 8.1. Kidney. There are some residual nuclei of the tubules and glomeruli (arrows).

Figure 8.2. Kidney. In this higher-power image the loss of basophilia of tubular and glomerular nuclei is easily seen.

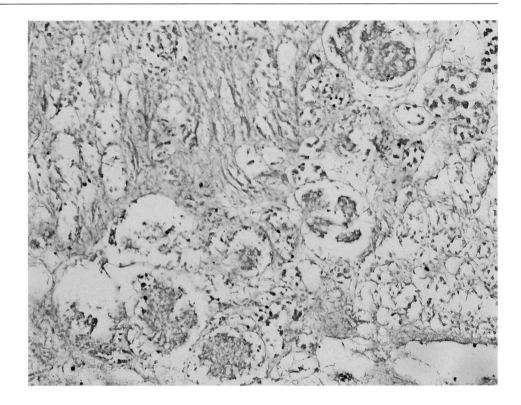

Figure 8.3. Adrenal gland. There is loss of nuclear basophilia involving the entire organ. The arrow marks the cortex and the asterisk identifies the medulla.

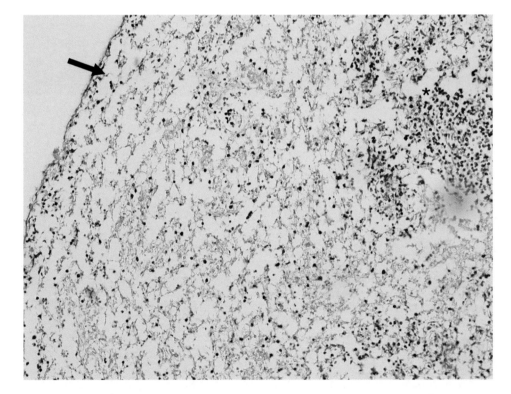

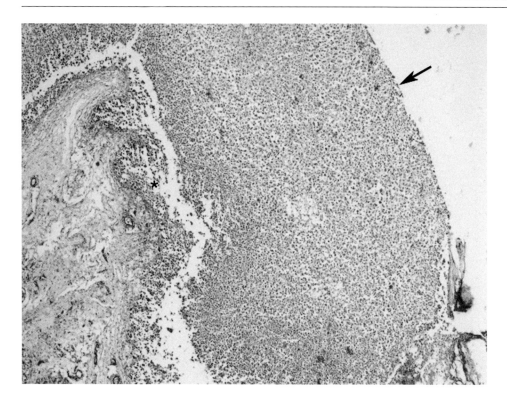

Figure 8.4. Adrenal gland. A lower-power view demonstrates the loss of nuclear staining of the adrenal cortex.

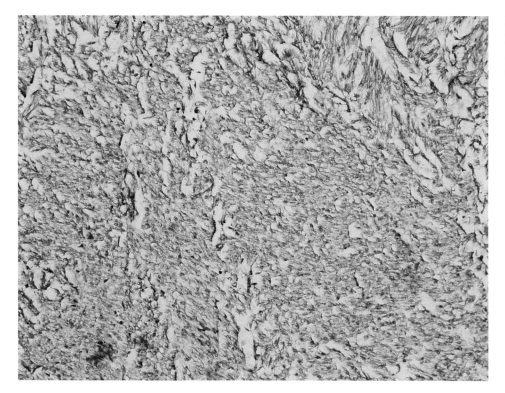

Figure 8.5. Heart. There is loss of nuclear staining of the cardiac myocytes just beneath the endocardium.

Figure 8.6. Liver. There is focal loss of nuclei with some preservation of surrounding parenchyma (arrows).

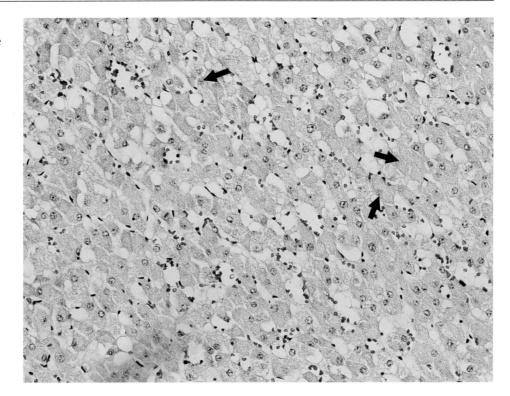

Figure 8.7. Lung. There is loss of nuclear basophilia of the alveolar epithelial cells (arrows).

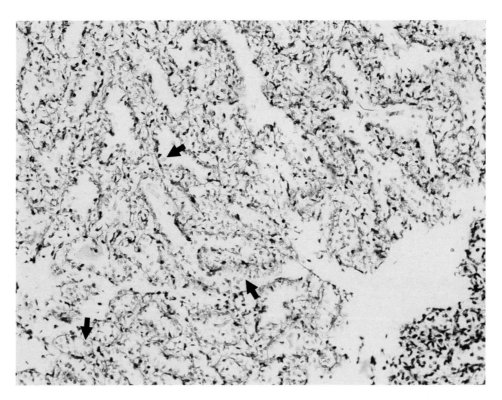

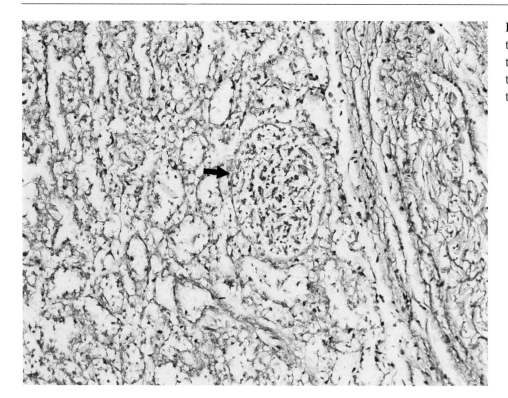

Figure 8.8. Lung. In addition to loss of nuclear staining of the alveolar epithelial cells, there is also degeneration of the bronchiole (arrow).

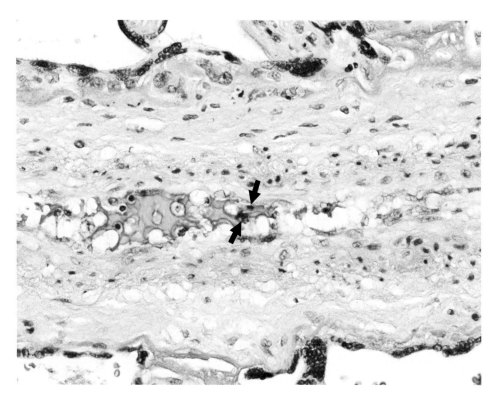

Figure 8.9A, B, C. Placenta. There is multifocal karyorrhexis of intraluminal leukocytes (Figures 8.9A, B: arrows) and fibrous luminal obliteration (Figure 8.9 C,: between arrows).

Figure 8.9B.

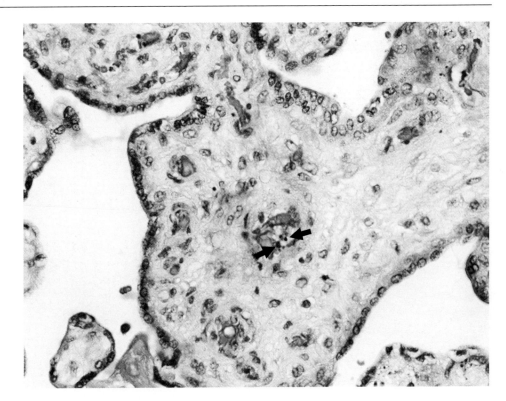

Figure 8.9C.

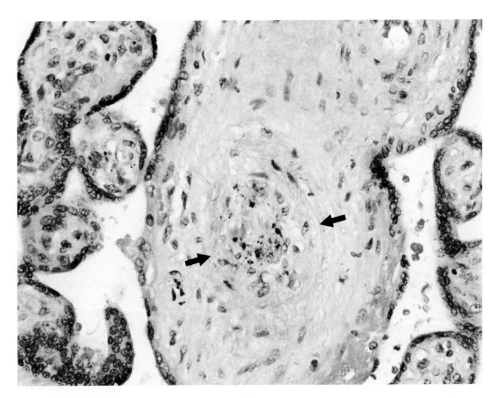

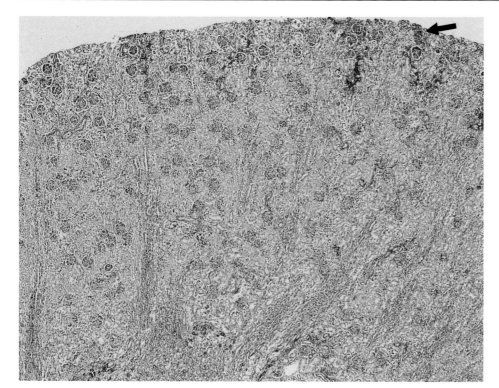

Figure 8.10A. Normal infant kidney. There is a residual germinal layer present (arrow) that may remain for up to 12 months of age.

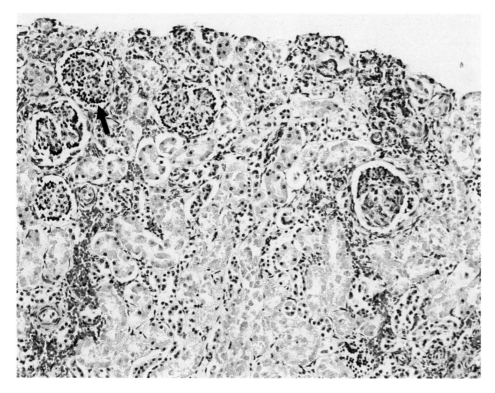

Figure 8.10B. A higher-power view of the normal infant kidney. Notice the rim of hyperchromatic nuclei surrounding the glomeruli (arrow), typical of glomeruli in the germinal layer.

Figure 8.11. A high-power view of a normal infant kidney. The glomeruli are slightly hypercellular with a rim of hyperchromatic nuclei (arrowhead). Rare sclerotic glomeruli are also present, often close to the cortex, and represent a normal finding (arrow).

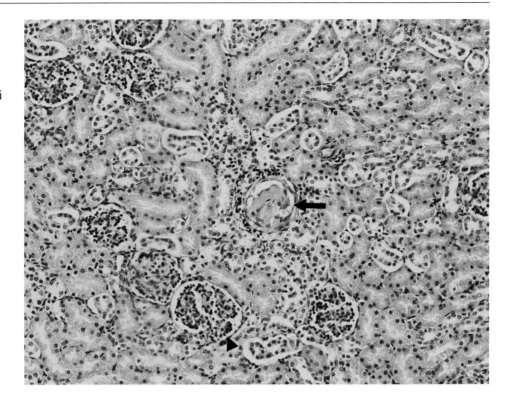

Figure 8.12. Normal infant lung. Infant lung demonstrates a more cellular interstitium. There should be at least four alveoli between the pleural surface (arrow) and the most distal bronchiole.

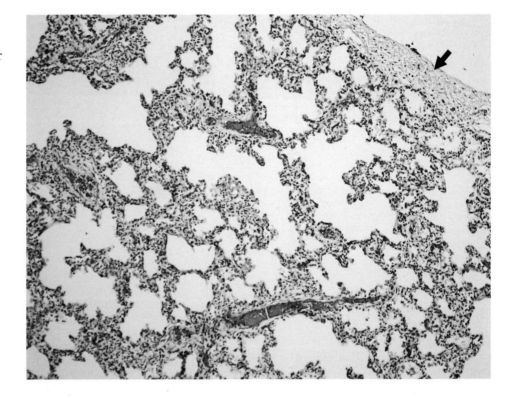

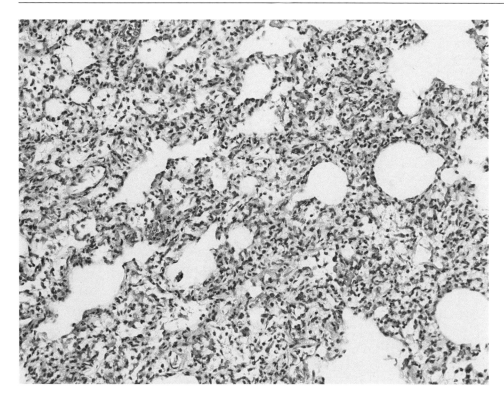

Figure 8.13. Atelectatic infant lung. Quite frequently an infant lung is atelectatic under the microscope. When this occurs it is easy to confuse with the increased cellularity commonly associated with inflammatory changes. One approach that is helpful is to identify the bronchi or bronchioles. In viral infection there is typically increased inflammation around these structures.

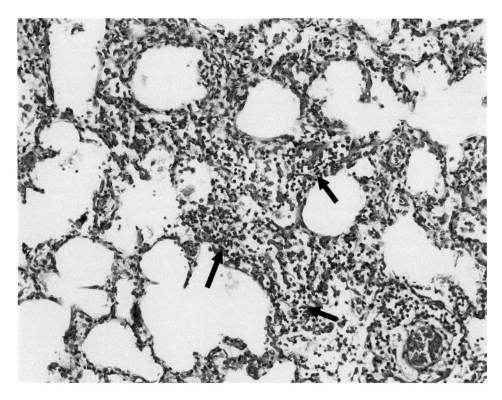

Figure 8.14. Viral lung. There is a chronic inflammatory infiltrate within the alveolar septae in conjunction with edema (arrows). The septae appear widened as a result of this reaction. Also note the perivascular edema.

Figure 8.15. Glial–neuronal heterotopia of the leptomeninges. There is an ectopic neuron (arrow) within the leptomeninges in this section of pons from a 4-month-old infant. Though non-specific, this finding has been associated with Sudden Infant Death Syndrome (SIDS).

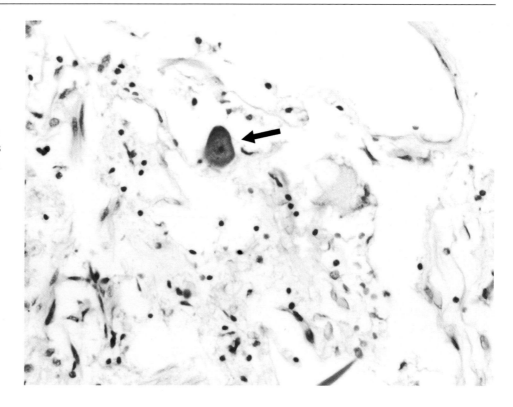

INFLICTED INJURY

A few words about radiology and injury

In most cases it is impossible to differentiate accidental from non-accidental injuries on radiological grounds. The use of radiology to detect injuries is fraught with problems and there is variability in the ability for radiology to detect injury in different anatomic locations (Evans, 1981). In regards to skull fractures, the positive predictive value of CT (computerised tomography) to detect all skull fractures is 72%, as found in a study by Molina and DiMaio (2008). The positive predictive value of detecting occipital bone fractures is 37.5%. In this same study the positive predictive value of detecting rib fractures was 83.5%; liver injury 50%; splenic injury 42.9%, and solid organ injury (pancreas, kidney, liver and spleen) was 43.8%. This study was conducted on adults, so application to children must be done with some caution; however, it must be noted that detecting injury by radiology in the case of children may be problematic and it is always wise to perform the autopsy and "see the injury with your own eyes" instead of relying on radiology reports.

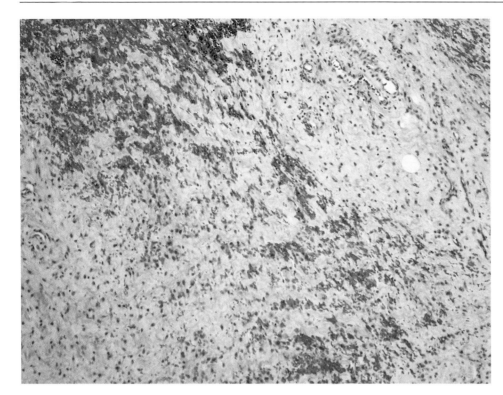

Figure 8.16. Retroperitoneal hemorrhage. There is acute hemorrhage within the retroperitoneal soft tissue. In cases of abuse these injuries are consistent with blunt impacts to the abdomen, such as stomps, kicks, or punches. It is important always to sample the retroperitoneal tissue in suspected abuse cases as it is common for the child to have been abused previously ("battered child syndrome") and residual chronic inflammation and fibrosis may be found in such instances.

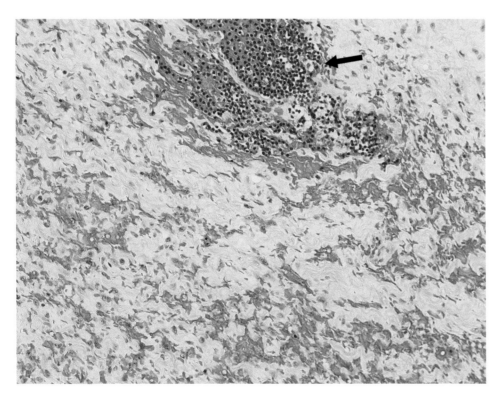

Figure 8.17. Retroperitoneal hemorrhage. One must remember that the retroperitoneal tissue is rich in lymphoid tissue (arrow) and these normal lymphoid structures should not be confused with chronic inflammation.

Figure 8.18. Retroperitoneal hemorrhage. There are focal macrophages present adjacent to the areas of acute hemorrhage (arrow).

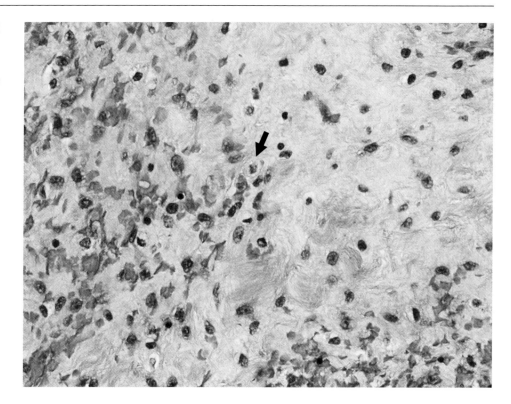

A few words about axonal injury

A few words about amyloid precursor protein (APP). Interpretation of APP stains can be challenging. Not all that decorates is diffuse axonal injury! Multiple papers have been published describing many different types of axonal injury (see "Suggested reading" section). Of forensic interest are traumatic axonal injury and hypoxic/ischemic axonal injury. Traumatic axonal injury is caused by direct trauma to the axon and typically results in balls or clumps of positive APP staining (Figure 8.20A, B, C). Hypoxic/ischemic axonal injury results in a less obvious staining pattern of delicate strands of APP-positive axons that resemble zebra skin (Figure 8.21A and B). One must use caution when reading APP-stained slides and learn to recognize the different patterns. This is particularly true with children, where positive APP staining DOES NOT diagnose "shaken-impact" syndrome! Any child with a head injury that results in hypoxia will have positive APP stains. Again, positive APP is not diagnostic of child abuse! This is a useful stain if used properly. It is also quite useful in that, according to most published papers, positive staining can be seen as early as 90 minutes post insult.

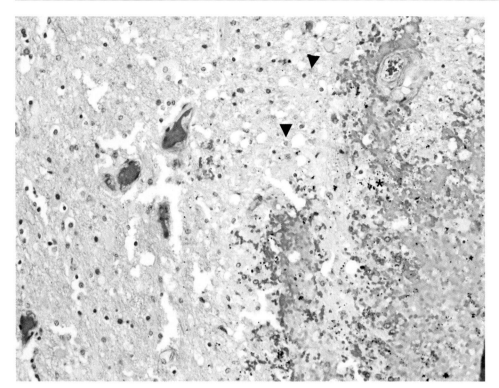

Figure 8.19. Axonal injury. There is acute hemorrhage surrounded by necrotizing brain parenchyma. Rare axonal retraction balls are seen on this haematoxylin and eosin (H&E) stain (arrowheads). It is difficult to identify axonal retraction balls by H&E before 24 hours. Notice the degenerating red-appearing neurons and edema. The red blood cells are beginning to lose their cytoplasmic borders. The age of this lesion can be estimated at 3 to 5 days. The dark granular material (asterisk) is formalin pigment and should not be confused with hemosiderin.

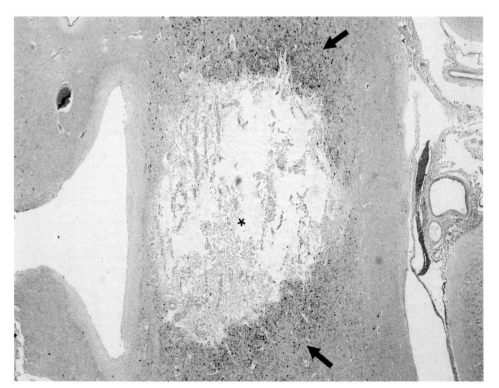

Figure 8.20A. Amyloid precursor protein (APP) immunohistochemistry. A section of corpus callosum stained with APP, demonstrating axonal retraction balls (arrows). There is a large cavity filled with macrophages (asterisk). This 6-month-old infant died as the result of admitted shaking.

Figure 8.20B and C. Higher magnification of the lesion.

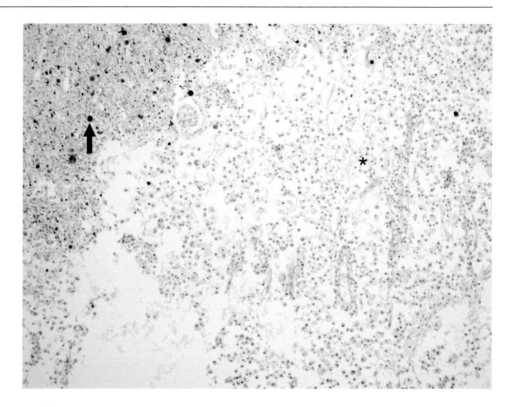

Figure 8.20C.

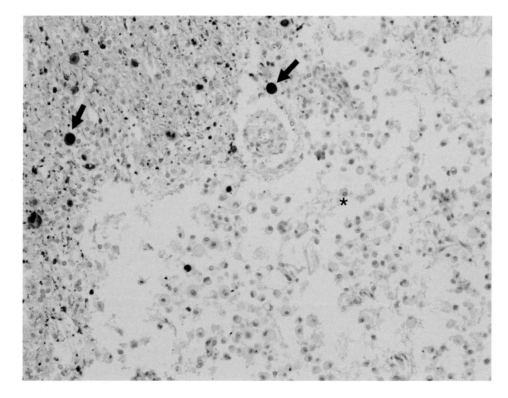

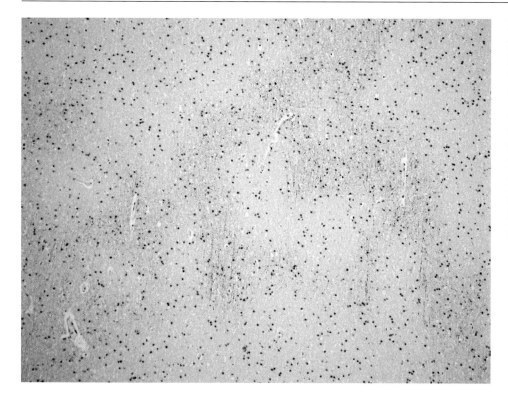

Figure 8.21A. Amyloid precursor protein (APP) immunohistochemical stain. This APP stain demonstrates the subtle, delicate staining seen with hypoxia. Notice the strands of positive-staining axons throughout the section. Take a step back and look from a distance – it is quite obvious! It has been termed hypoxic/ischemic or vascular axonal injury.

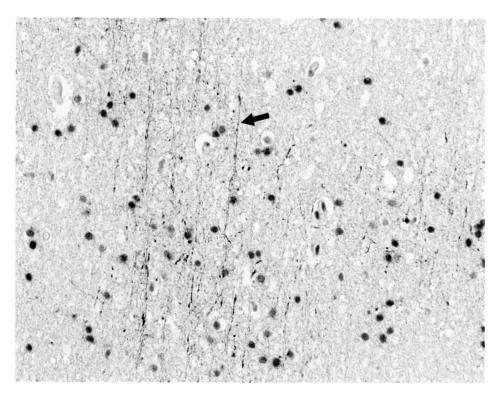

Figure 8.21B. Amyloid precursor protein (APP) immunohistochemical stain. This is a higher-power view of Figure 8.21A. Notice the long strand of positive APP staining (arrow).

FRACTURE DATING

Figure 8.22. Skull. There is an acute fracture (arrow) of the skull with acute hemorrhage (asterisk). The red blood cells are intact and there is fibrin deposition. This section was placed in decalcification solution, which may account for the pallor of the red blood cells.

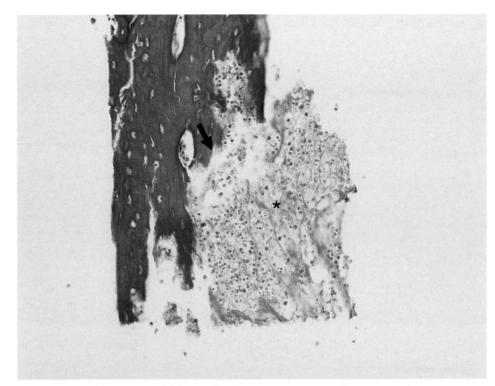

Figure 8.23. Normal rib of a two-year-old child demonstrating thick bony spicules (asterisks), sparse marrow cavity, and periosteal soft tissue (arrowheads). Depending on the region of the rib for study, there may be more or less marrow cavity.

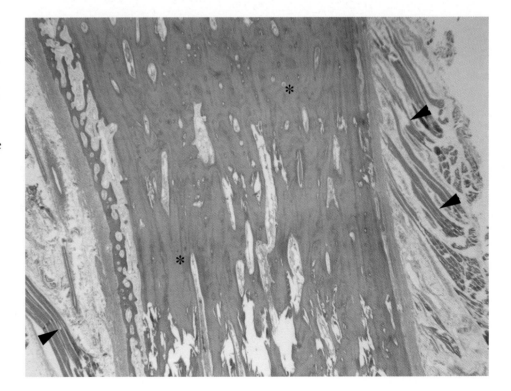

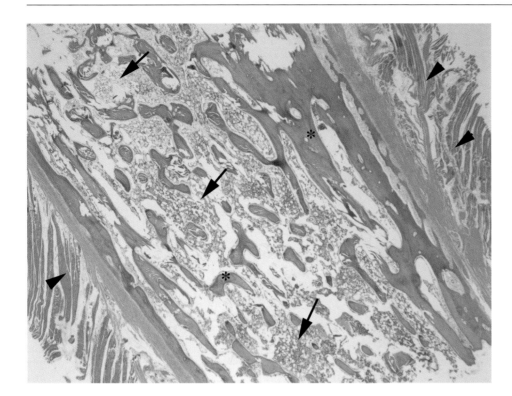

Figure 8.24. Normal rib of a two-year-old child demonstrating bony spicules (asterisks), marrow cavity (arrows), and periosteal soft tissue. Depending on the region of the rib for study, there may be more or less marrow cavity.

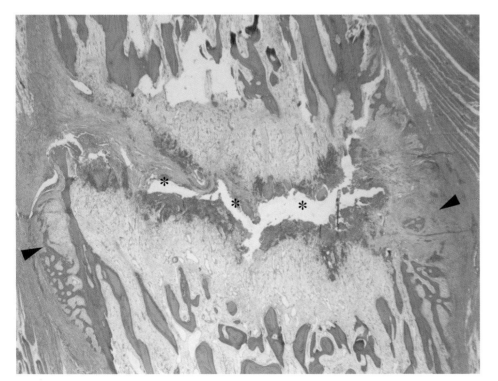

Figure 8.25. Subacute fracture (approximately day 7–10 post-fracture) with acute hemorrhage, fibrin, trabecular bone fragments, and early granulation tissue in the fracture gap (asterisks). Note the early callus formation comprised of cartilage and new bone at the periphery of the fracture gap (arrowheads).

Figure 8.26. Higher-power view of the fracture gap.

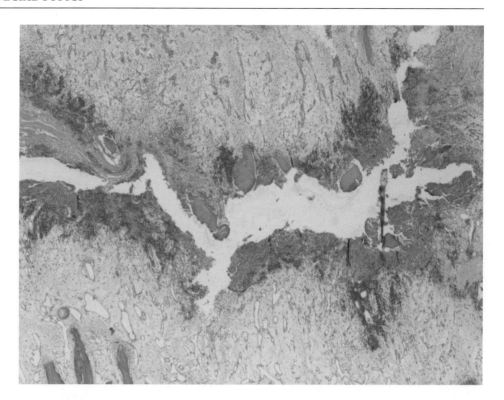

Figure 8.27. Higher-power views of the early periosteal callus comprised of cartilage proliferation (arrowhead) and new bone formation (arrows).

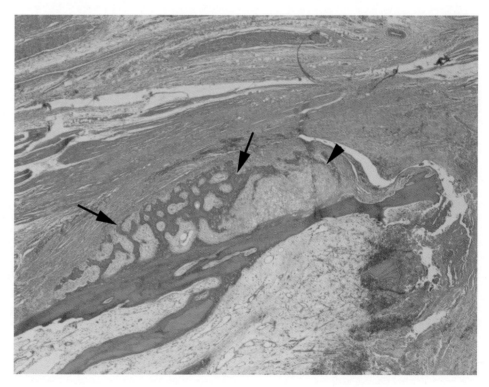

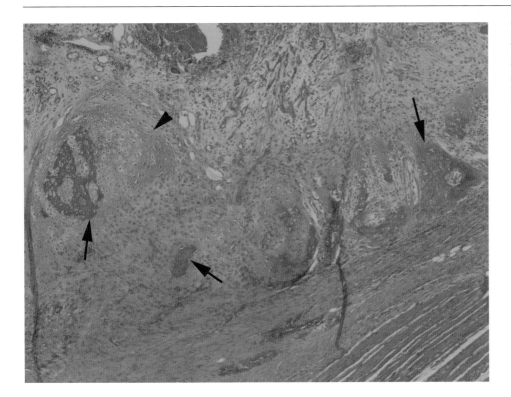

Figure 8.28. Higher-power views of the early periosteal callus comprised of cartilage proliferation (arrowhead) and new bone formation (arrows).

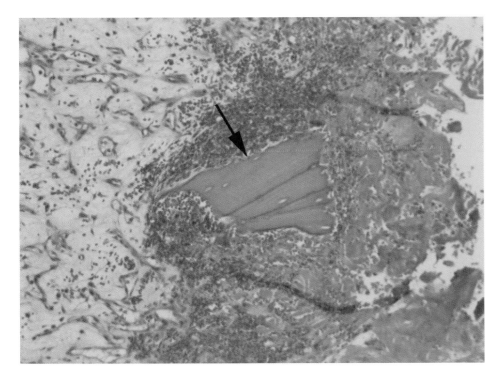

Figure 8.29. High-power view of necrotic bone in the subacute fracture gap with surrounding hemorrhage (arrow). Note the lack of osteocytes in the lacunae of the bone fragment.

Figure 8.30. Osteoclasts have moved in and are resorbing old bone near the fracture gap.

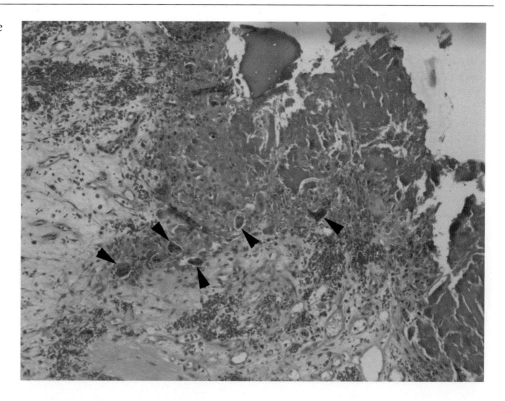

Figure 8.31. Later in fracture healing, the callus has evolved with cartilage in-growth (arrowheads) into the fracture gap, ossification, and new bone is being formed (arrows).

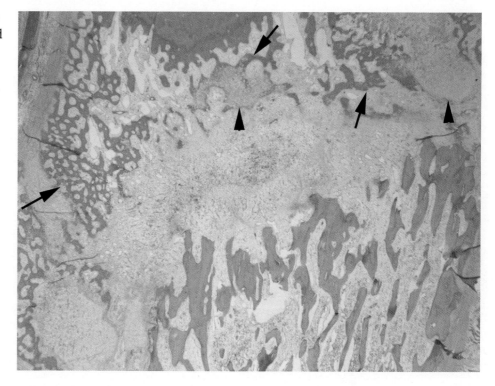

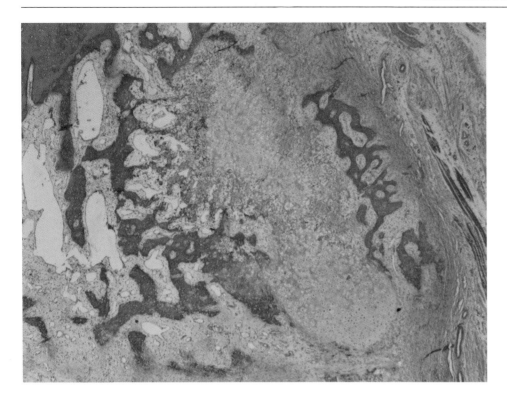

Figure 8.32. Periosteal callus comprised of cartilage with peripheral new bone formation and ossification.

It must be noted that histologic dating of infant rib fractures must be correlated with the investigative information available, the clinical history (if hospitalized), radiologic imaging (if available), and the metabolic and nutritional status of the child.

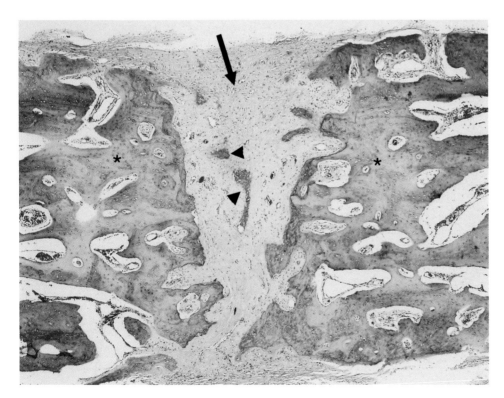

Figure 8.33. Skull suture. Notice the homogenous fibrovascular tissue (arrow) with delicate vasculature between areas of bone (asterisk). The suture is beginning to ossify as there are islands of newly forming bone within the fibrovascular tissue (arrowheads). There is no granulation tissue and there is no hemosiderin deposition, which helps differentiate the suture from a fracture. This section was taken from an anomalous parietal suture that was called a fracture on radiology.

Figure 8.33B. Skull suture. Higher-power view of the fibrovascular tissue (arrowheads).

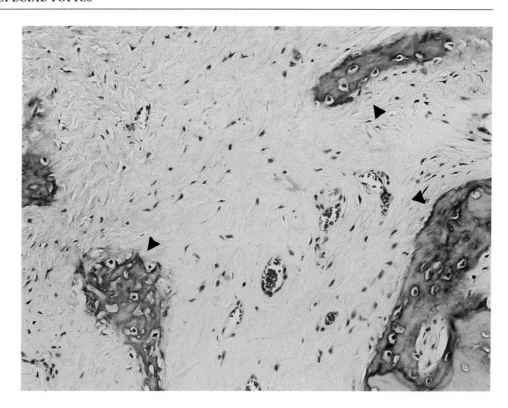

Table 8.2 Microscopic and radiologic landmarks in healing infant rib fractures.

Earliest appearance	Usual appearance	Landmark
24 hours	2–3 days	RAD: Periosteal thickening MIC: Initial acute hemorrhage in fracture cavity and proliferation of fibroblastic, chondrocytic, and osteogenic cells from the periosteum and endosteum
4–5 days	7–14 days	RAD: Obvious callus and first formation of new bone MIC: Osteoblastic, osteoclastic, chondroblastic, and fibroblastic proliferation with angiogenesis (callus formation) and subsequent formation of new bone
2–3 weeks	3–6 weeks	MIC: Bony union of fracture

MIC = microscopic; RAD= radiographic.

Remember that these observations represent a continuum of changes and must be taken in to consideration in light of the clinical history and general health of the infant involved.

Callus exuberance and the progress of healing are dependent upon the degree of fracture displacement after injury, immobilization of fractured ends during healing, the integrity of the periosteum and surrounding soft tissue, and the nutritional status of the infant.

By virtue of actively growing bones, infants and children heal more quickly than adults.

Source:

Zumwalt, R.E. and Fanizza-Orphanos, A.M. Dating of healing rib fractures in fatal child abuse. *Adv. Pathol* (1990), **3**, 193–205.

A few words about retinal hemorrhages

The significance of retinal hemorrhage and optic nerve sheath hemorrhage is controversial. These hemorrhages are not, in and of themselves, sufficient to determine the presence of inflicted injury. Other circumstances under which retinal and optic nerve sheath hemorrhages may be found include resuscitation and cerebral edema. A recent retrospective study (Matshes, 2010) of 123 autopsies of children up to 3 years old showed retinal hemorrhage, optic nerve sheath hemorrhage, or both, in 18 cases. Of these, two were certified as natural deaths, eight as accidents, and eight as homicides. One finding of note was hemorrhage in six of seven cases without any head injury. There is a widespread belief among clinicians that skull fractures, subdural hematomas, and retinal hemorrhages do not occur in accidental short falls. In reality, all three have been found in cases of falls from short heights.

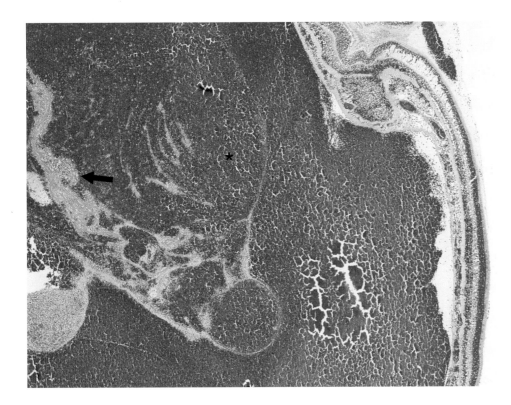

Figure 8.34A. Retinal hemorrhages. There is acute hemorrhage within the vitreous (asterisk) with focal areas of acute inflammation and fibrin deposition (arrow). There is also acute hemorrhage within the retinal tissue.

Figure 8.34B and C. Retinal hemorrhages. There is acute hemorrhage within the retinal tissue.

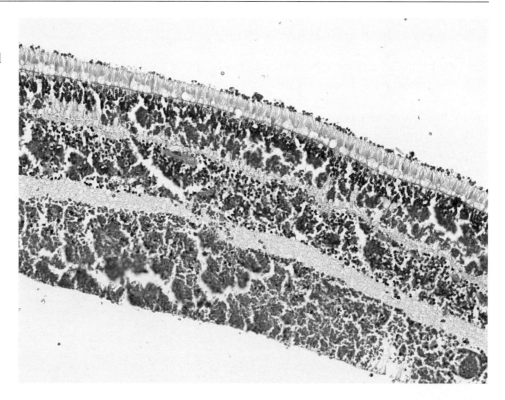

Figure 8.34C.

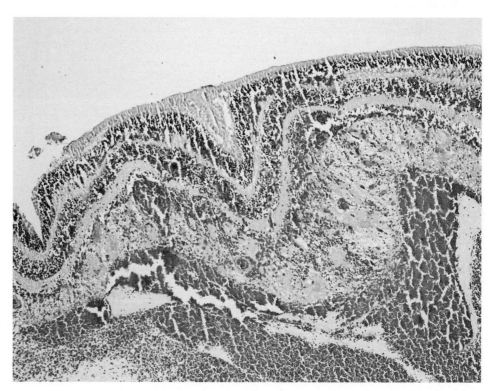

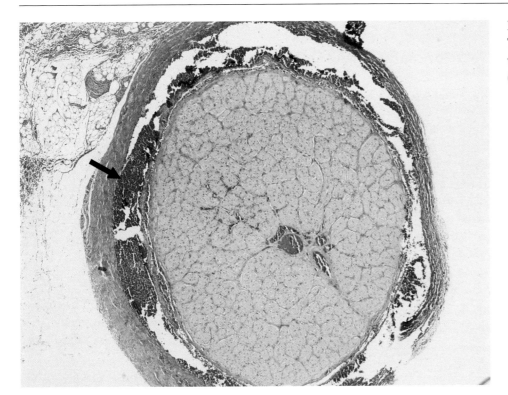

Figure 8.35A. Optic nerve. There is acute hemorrhage within the optic nerve sheath (arrow).

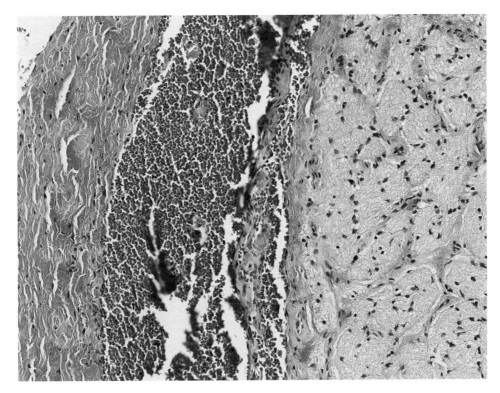

Figure 8.35B. Optic nerve. A higher-power view showing acute hemorrhage between the sheath and the optic nerve.

Not to be confused with skin contusions

Figure 8.36A. Mongolian spot. These may be confused with contusions. They are congenital pigmented lesions (nevi) that are usually found on the buttocks or backs of darkly pigmented infants. Upon incising these lesions, there is no subcutaneous hemorrhage. Microscopically, there are dermal melanocytes. (Photograph courtesy of Steven Cina, Ft. Lauderdale, FL.)

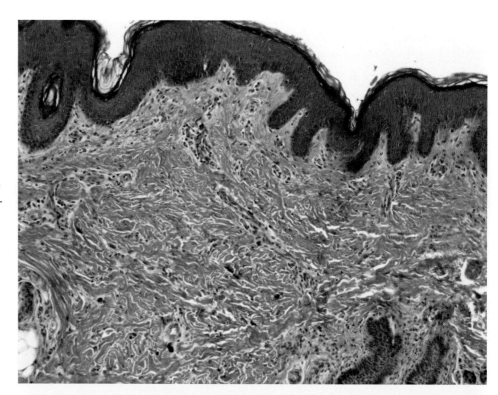

Figure 8.36B. Mongolian spot. Higher power showing dermal melanocytes. (Photograph courtesy of Steven Cina, Ft. Lauderdale, FL.)

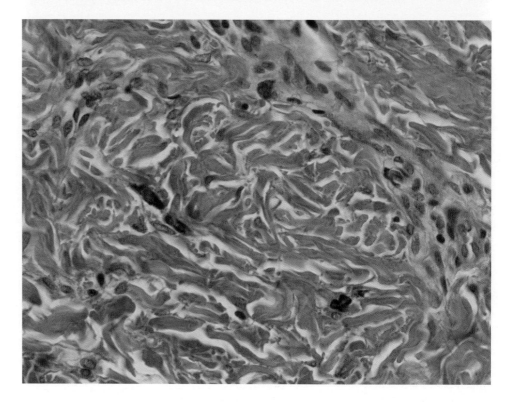

SUGGESTED READING

Inflicted versus accidental injury

Berney, J., Froidevaux, A.C., Favier, J . Paediatric head trauma: influence of age and sex: II. Biomechanical and anatomo-clinical correlations. *Childs Nerv Syst.* 1994; **10**: 517–523.

Croft, P.R., Reichard, R.R. Microscopic examination of grossly unremarkable pediatric dura mater. *Am J Forensic Med Pathol.* 2009; **30**(1): 10–13.

Dedouit, F., Guilbeau-Frugier, C., Capuani, C., Sevely, A., *et al.* Child abuse: practical applications of autopsy, radiological, and microscopic studies. *J Forensic Sci.* 2008; **53**(6): 1424–1429.

Denton, S., Mileusnic, D. Delayed sudden death in an infant following an accidental fall: A case report with review of the liteature. *Am J Forensic Med Pathol.* 2003; **24**(4): 371–376.

Duhaime AC, Alario AJ, Lewander WJ, *et al.* Head injury in very young children: mechanisms, injury types, and opthalmologic findings in 100 hospitalized patients younger than 2 years of age. *Pediatrics.* 1992; **90**(2): 179–186.

Duhaime, A.C., Christian, C.W., Rorke, L.B., Zimmerman, R. Nonaccidental head injury in infants – the "shaken baby syndrome". *NEJM.*1998; **338**(25): 1823–1829.

Dye, D.W., Peretti, F.J., Kokes, C.P. Histologic evidence of repetitive blunt force abdominal trauma in four pediatric fatalities. *J Forensic Sci.* 2008; **53**(6): 1430–1433.

Evans, K.T., Knight, B. *Forensic Radiology.* Oxford: Blackwell Scientific Publications, 1981.

Ewing-Cobbs, L., Kramer, L., Prasad, M., *et al.* Neuroimaging, physical, and developmental findings after inflicted and non-inflicted traumatic brain injury in young children. *Pediatrics.* 1998; **102**(2): 300–307.

Fenton, L.Z., Sirotnak, A.P., Handler, M.H. Parietal pseudofracture and spontaneous intracranial hemorrhage suggesting non-accidental trauma: report of 2 cases. *Pediatr Neurosurg.* 2000; **33**: 318–322.

Geddes, J.F., Hackshaw, A.K., Vowles, G.H., Nickols, C.D., Whitwell, H.L. Neuropathology of inflicted head injury in children: I. Patterns of brain damage. *Brain.* 2001; **124**: 1290–1298.

Geddes, J.F., Vowles, G.H., Hackshaw, A.K., Nickols, C.D., Whitwell, H.L. Neuropathology of inflicted head injury in children: II. Microscopic brain injury in infants. *Brain.* 2001; **124**: 1299–1306.

Genest, D.R., Williams, M.A., Greene, M.F. Estimating the time of death in stillborn fetuses: I. Histologic evaluation of fetal organs – an autopsy study of 150 stillborns. *Obstet Gynaecol.* 1992; **80**(4): 575–599.

Gill, J.R., Goldfeder, L.B., Armbrustmacher, V., et al. Fatal head injury in children younger than 2 years in New York City and an overview of the shaken baby syndrome. *Arch Pathol Lab Med.* 2009; **133**: 619–627.

Lantz, P.E., Couture, D.E. Fatal acute intracranial injury with subdural hematoma and retinal hemorrhages in an infant due to stairway fall. *American Academy of Forensic Sciences Proceedings*, **16**, 2010.

Lantz, P.E., Sinal, S.H., Stanton, C.A., Weaver, R.G., Jr. Perimacular retinal folds from childhood head trauma. *BMJ.* 2004; **328**(7442): 754–756.

Matshes, E. Retinal and optic nerve sheath hemorrhages are not pathognomonic of abusive head injury. *American Academy of Forensic Sciences Proceedings*, **16**, 2010.

Molina, D.K., DiMaio, V.J. The sensitivity of computerised tomography (CT) scans in detecting trauma: are CT scans reliable enough for courtroom testimony? *Trauma*. 2008; **65**(5): 1206–1207.

Oehmichen, M., Schleiss, D., Pedal, I., *et al.* Shaken baby syndrome: re-examination of diffuse axonal injury as a cause of death. *Acta Neuropathol.*2008; **116**: 317–329.

Plunkett, J. Fatal pediatric head injuries cause by short distance falls. *Am J Forensic Med Pathol*. 2001; **22**(1): 1–12.

Reichard, R.R., White, C.L., Hladik, C.L., Dolinak, D. Beta-amyolid precursor protein staining of non-accidental central nervous system injury in pediatric autopsies. *J Neurotrauma*. 2003; **20**(4): 347–355.

Root, I. Head injuries from short distance falls. *Am J Forensic Med Pathol*. 1992; **13**(1): 85–87.

Sauvageau, A., Bourgault, A., Racette, S. Cerebral traumatism with a playground rocking toy mimicking shaken baby syndrome. *J Forensic Sci*. 2008; **53**(2): 479–82.

Squire W. Shaken baby syndrome: the quest for evidence. *Dev Med Child Neurol*. 2008; **50**: 10–14.

Natural or undetermined causes of death

Machaalani, R., Say, M., Waters, KA. Serotoninergic receptor 1A in the sudden infant death syndrome brainstem medulla and associations with clinical risk factors. *Acta Neuropathol*. 2009; **117**: 257–265.

Figure 5.14C 2.

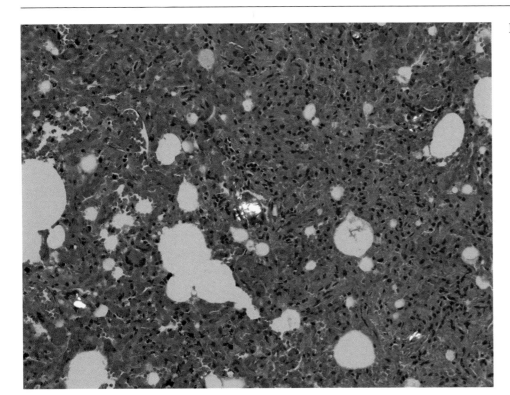

Figure 5.14C 3.

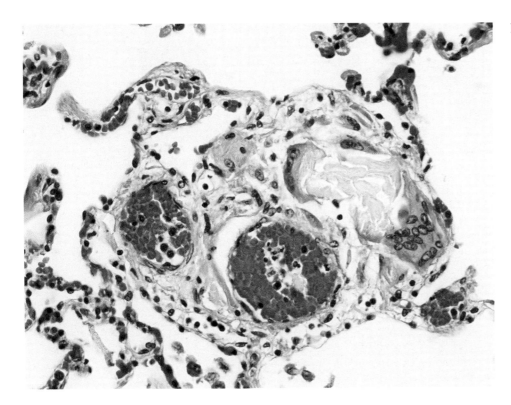

Figure 5.14C 4

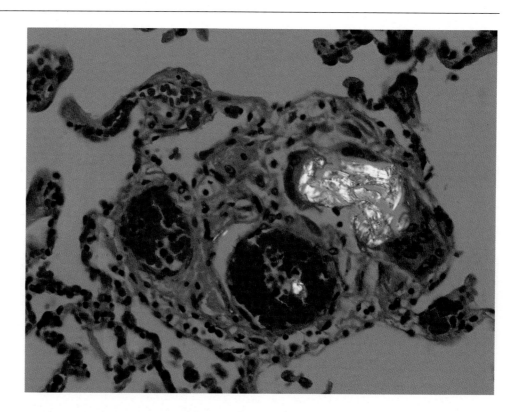

Figure 5.15A. Cutaneous injection site. Low-power view with acute hemorrhage into the subdermal adipose tissue (arrow) and assembly of foreign body-type giant cells (arrowheads).

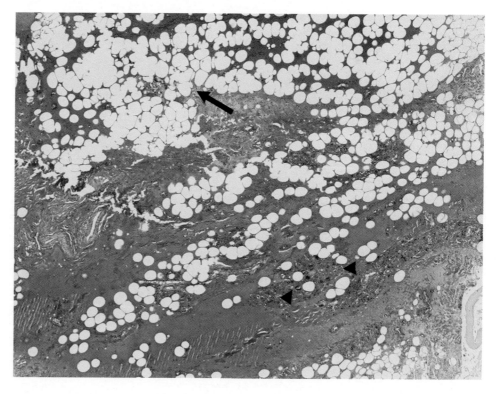

INDEX